D1649932

Relief from Pain with
Finger Massage

Relief from Pain with Finger Massage

Dr Roger Dalet

Translated by Linda Zuck

Hutchinson of London

Hutchinson & Co. (Publishers) Ltd
3 Fitzroy Square, London W1P 6JD

London Melbourne Sydney Auckland
Wellington Johannesburg Cape Town
and agencies throughout the world

First published in Great Britain 1979

©Opera Mundi, Paris 1978
Translation © Hutchinson Publishing Group 1979

Printed in Great Britain by
MᶜCorquodale (Newton) Ltd., Newton-le-Willows, Lancashire

British Library CIP data
Dalet, Roger
  Finger massage.
  1. Acupressure
  I. Title
  615¹.822   RM723.A27

ISBN 0 09 139501 1

Contents

Introduction

Although we traditionally speak only of five senses – touch, taste, smell, hearing and sight – there is a sixth sensation which is the most severe and disturbing, and which demands attention and relief: *pain*. Yet, paradoxically, while most of us would regard pain as totally evil, it is also an important survival mechanism, as those very few people who are born without the ability to perceive pain know to their cost; they continually suffer injury, in circumstances where the rest of us would have received warning signals of danger, either from outside ourselves, or from internal disease processes.

So pain has a survival value and should be attended to as soon as it occurs, generally by seeking skilled medical attention. But pain often, if not usually, has disadvantages which far outweigh the benefits. Having served its warning purpose it outstays its welcome; or sometimes the warning has been a false alarm; or the signal gives a quite disproportionately exaggerated indication of the underlying cause, which may be trivial. Such pain may be disabling while serving no purpose, and it is pain such as this that we are aiming to treat in this book.

Everyone, these days, has heard of acupuncture. Until recently we tended to think of it as a secret, very mysterious, and very complicated oriental method of medical treatment. But with the opening up of China to foreign visitors, many reports have now emerged of major surgical operations being performed under acupuncture anaesthesia alone, and of the use of acupuncture to treat a wide variety of conditions, even some, such as deafness, which are not particularly associated with pain. Films of this treatment have been shown on television, and reports have been published in the serious scientific medical journals of Europe and America.

In China itself, thousands of men and women, the so-called 'barefoot doctors', have been trained to look after, relieve, or cure the complaints and ailments of their own families, their neighbours, and their fellow workers, and to do this simply by stimulating certain selected points on the body.

Anyone can learn to relieve his own aches and pains, and those of his children, friends and neighbours, by the same methods. We are not talking here about the full system of acupuncture treatment. This is the province of the professional acupuncturists, who have been studying and perfecting the method for years. We are talking, rather, about a method of obtaining quick, even if sometimes only temporary, relief, a method simpler to apply, but based on exactly the same principles as acupuncture; a method, which is at least as effective as taking pills or medicine, for the relief of such complaints as lumbago, which makes you double up with excruciating pain, or all those other troublesome aches; but this method also can be used to cure some complaints – not especially painful, but disturbing –such as insomnia.

Historical background

Traditional methods of treatment in Chinese medicine, whether using needles or the application of heat, go back to the beginning of time.

Current excavation of prehistoric tombs, which date back to the period before the invention of writing, is turning up, indeed more and more often, needles which were undoubtedly used for therapeutic purposes. Often these needles are simply splinters chipped from small pointed stones or flints, but gold and silver needles, somewhat oxidized over the years, have been found in the tombs of nobles and kings, and in the sarcophagai of princes and princesses.

There are, of course, very few original documents relating to the origins of the ancient science of acupuncture, and this is why there is an abundance of hypotheses about the beginnings of this practice; there are even people who think that the origins and growth of this method of medicine, so peculiar to China, may be explained by a visit from outer space. But without going quite so far, one can — we think — willingly accept that the reports of scrupulously careful and critical observers from the West, at the invitation of the Chinese, have allowed this whole important structure, which is for us a new, and, on the surface of it, strange, system of medicine, to be brought to Western consciousness.

Early in the history of China people were trying to systematize the practice of acupuncture. As early as 220 BC, an important work called the *Nei-King, Nei-Jing,* or *Nei-Ching,* was commissioned by the Emperor Houang-Ti, the 'Yellow Emperor'. He wrote in one of his edicts: "I am disturbed by the amounts in taxes and dues that do not reach me on account of illness amongst the people. My wish is that we should no longer use medicine, which poisons them, or ancient methods. I want those mysterious metal needles, which direct energy, to be used instead."

The whole of acupuncture rests on this phrase, and over the succeeding centuries, careful, patient and repeated observations have allowed the method in all its aspects to be defined.

The practice flourished, and was widely used and taught. Around AD 1400 the bronze statuette known as the bronze man, a statue pierced with holes corresponding to the acupuncture points on the skin, was being used as a model to teach students.

The use of acupuncture only suffered an eclipse relatively recently, when towards the beginning of the nineteenth century invading Europeans, with their distrust of traditional medicine, influenced the élites of Chinese society to introduce the methods of Western medicine. In particular, during the last years of the government which preceeded the present régime in China, traditional medicine was outlawed, and was only able to survive in remote country areas. It was not until Mao Tse-tung came to power that traditional medicine was generally reinstated, and it came to be both practised and taught in hospitals, as well as in workplaces where 'barefoot doctors' could treat their fellow workers.

Today, medical research and therapeutics in China is more or less equally split between traditional and Western methods, as Mao Tse-tung had wished.

The underlying theory of acupuncture is complex, but the main principles are clearly defined. Here we shall describe them, and use them as a skeleton for as much additional theory as is necessary.

Above all, acupuncture is a philosophy, or rather a method of treatment that has been incorporated into the Chinese cosmological and philosophical tradition. In classical Chinese thought, the world of matter and the world of energy are a continuity. We can draw a striking parallel between this binary system and that defined in the West by Einstein and his followers.

In the Chinese tradition the two elements of this binary system are called Yin and Yang; they symbolize the light and dark aspects of things, and these two forces completely complement each other, and merge into one another without disturbing each other, as inevitably as day follows night, and ice becomes water. They are, in short, two aspects or sides of the same truth.

This binary system underlies the whole structure and functioning of matter, and matter, according to the Chinese, is composed of five different elements. Numbers were very important in ancient Chinese philosophy – after all, it was they who, through the Persians and the Arabs, gave us our present system of numbers, and the number five was particularly significant to them.

So, there were five cardinal points (the Chinese add the centre to the four that we describe), five planets, five tastes, five smells, and there are also five elements, earth, fire, water, air and wood; and each of these five elements was held to correspond with one of our specific organs. And all of this intermingles, through a network of correspondences. It is as if the ancient Chinese philosophers had discovered the French poet Baudelaire's famous phrase: *"Les parfums, les couleurs et les sons se répondent"**

But it is also interesting that ancient Greek – and indeed Western medicine until relatively modern times – was based on the very similar system of the four elements: earth, air, fire, and water; the four properties: hot, cold, wet, and dry; and the four humours: blood, phlegm, yellow bile and black bile. The humours were believed to correspond not only to the appropriate mixture of these elements and properties, but also to the seasons of the year, and the temperaments and dispositions of individual people. So there was in earlier times a link between the foundations on which Chinese and Western medical theory rested.

But acupuncture is not only philosophical theory, it is also a system of medicine and a technique of treatment. It is always interesting to see the completely different ways in which traditional Chinese doctors work in the operating theatre, as compared with Western doctors. Of course the Chinese doctor makes a diagnosis; but to do this, he uses elements which are disregarded by Western doctors. He examines carefully the patient's face, his expression, the colour of his eyes, the colour and grain of his skin; he carefully examines, quite literally millimetre by millimetre, the patient's tongue; and in so doing he discovers the correspondences with the central organs. He feels the abdomen, but not in the way that a Western doctor does who is looking for the size of the liver, spleen, and other organs, but very lightly and gently, stroking almost, each region of the abdominal wall. This tells him things about the workings of the organs, and about the person in general. And finally, above all, he takes the pulse.

In the West, although it may be felt in many of our arteries, we consider that we have only one pulse. In China, whether it be over the radial artery or any of the other peripheral arteries, it is thought that there are twelve pulses, corresponding to the organs, which are palpated with extreme sensitivity of touch, an extraordinary skill from which the acupuncturist gains a wealth of knowledge.

The Chinese doctor then moves on to therapy. The important thing to understand about the application of his therapeutic rules is that according to the Chinese conception, vital energy flows constantly throughout the body; in health this energy is made up of a balanced mixture of the Yin and Yang. There is a continuous flow of this vital energy both over the entire surface of the body, and along the special lines or channels which

*"The smells, colours and sounds commune with one another" – from Baudelaire's famous sonnet *Correspondances,* in the *Fleurs du Mal.*

correspond with the major organs. There is thus a line, which we in the West call a meridian, which corresponds with the heart, another with the lungs, another with the liver, and others with the spleen, kidneys, the small and large intestines, the bile ducts, the bladder and the stomach. There are other meridians which correspond to other functions. Finally, there are supplementary or connecting meridians which link all the main vessels together into a complex network.

If energy stops flowing, in other words if there is an obstruction somewhere along one of these meridians or if there is an imbalance of the proportions of the Yin and the Yang, illness will develop, and, in the same way, from a qualitative point of view, if a perverse energy replaces the normal vital energy, again illness will result. Now along these meridians there are points – 361 in all, plus a few scattered separate ones-which allow the flow of energy to be modified both qualitatively and quantitatively. And once the doctor is well informed and documented about the patient through his oriental examination, he is able, according to complex rules called by poetic names such as Mother-Son Rule or Rule of the Five Elements, to place small needles in carefully and specifically chosen spots, so that the normal flow of qualitatively correct energy may re-establish itself, and as a result, good health will return.

When such theories were introduced to the West, they produced cries of shock and outrage, since they failed completely to correspond with any established anatomical or physiological observations; after all, very few people, even to this day, has actually observed these meridians with the naked eye; and this explains why, on the various occasions when Chinese medicine was introduced and re-introduced into the West, it soon fell into disrepute, and was finally abandoned, until very recently that is. In the sixteenth century the Benedictines, returning from China, first expounded the fundamentals of Chinese medicine and brought back acupuncture needles; but they only aroused sarcasm. Then, during the nineteenth century, medical authors such as the father of the great composer Berlioz, tried again to argue the advantages of the strange and new technique. But among the successes there were also failures, and accidents, and again the method was quickly disregarded and the theory dismissed. Not until the end of the nineteenth century, when lay observers, not doctors, such as the famous Soulié de Morant, who was French consul in China and who studied Chinese medicine and translated Chinese texts, did the practice again begin to spread into the West. The most recent introduction occurred during the last few years, but even today acupuncture arouses scepticism, and even hostility, amongst a number of Western therapists and research scientists. There is a mass of evidence of this incredulity and antagonism even from the greatest authorities, from whom we would expect a more open-minded attitude.

But alongside the doubters, there are those who have tried, and whose successful results have fired them with enthusiasm. So we may say that the debate is still open; and it still rages in the West, even though it has no real reason to, since traditional acupuncture, as it used to be practised and taught, has undergone considerable development and change, above all in its country of origin. This is for two reasons; we have seen that in modern China, under the drive and will of Mao Tse-tung, it was felt to be important to build a bridge between modern Western science and traditional Chinese. This was achieved in China on two levels.

In the first place, Chinese doctors have adopted Western methods, and adapted them where necessary to complement their own; and Western doctors have been amazed by the results. This association of techniques has taken place principally in the area of general care and hygiene in clinics and hospitals. But in the West we have seen a number of missions of doctors or other interested people particularly astonished to find themselves watching the amazing sight of surgery, without conventional anaesthesia, being performed on a patient where analgesia, that is to say absence of pain, is achieved simply by inserting a needle into a specific point in the body. In this way, patients have been filmed and interviewed during the course of their operations, people who, for example, were having a lung or part of the stomach removed, or mothers who were giving birth by Caeserian section, while still awake and fully conscious. This was something which was totally unbelievable until we were given visual proof. And, as we have seen, this system of medicine has been taught right down to the level of those called 'barefoot doctors'; even to factory workers, and farm labourers, who have learned how to use the needles and so can relieve the afflictions, however serious, of their fellow workers, neighbours and family. Now some of these 'barefoot doctors' have been encouraged to conduct their own research; thus, one of them, Tchao Pou Yu, has become a popular hero, since he has been successful in treating the deaf and dumb. This has opened new horizons to Westerners.

Secondly, Chinese doctors and scientists have also greatly improved on their acupunctural techniques. They have discovered effective new points; they have discovered new paths which complement the known existing ones, and which link up skin points to the major organs; and they have experimented with new methods, in particular with sending an electric current through the acupuncture needles. But above all, the contemporary Chinese have greatly simplified the use of acupuncture, through repeated experimentation during treatment and surgery; in particular, they have considerably reduced the number of points used for treating different complaints. Often one point alone is enough to cover an entire region, whatever the pathological condition. These developments have been very influential, since effective and safe treatment can now be given in the simplest of ways, and they have been reinforced by very recent and exciting discoveries made by physiologists in the West, which at last provide a scientific basis, acceptable to the Western tradition, for the use of acupuncture. This is described in the last section of this book.

In any case, whatever the way in which acupuncture works, by using all the knowledge now available, we can if not cure ourselves completely, at least relieve our complaints by the application of pressure on a small number of specific points.

In this book we are going to look at and describe the stimulation of these pressure points.

Techniques of use

Acupuncture points have been well known in China from the earliest times, and most of them are held to correspond to specific organs. Acupuncturists work by inserting needles of varying lengths at these points.

Certain points correspond to certain areas of the body, very specific areas. When they are stimulated, the corresponding area is being treated, and responds to the stimulation.

How do you actually apply the stimulation by this pressure? First, carefully locate the points, as described in the following pages: each point occupies only a very small area, approximately half a square millimetre.

The diagrams and explanations which follow will, it is hoped, allow you to locate them easily. Also, once they are located, you cannot mistake them since they are painful and highly sensitive areas, and the feeling is quite different from the surrounding tissues. There is a scientific reason for this, as will be described later.

Having located the points, you now have to stimulate them. The acupuncturist will of course insert his needle, but massaging the point can be almost as effective.

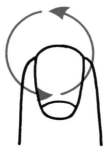

Place the tip of your index or second finger or thumb, on the point and press down forcefully, vibrating your finger slightly, or giving a rapid massage and rotating clockwise.

If you want to be even more precisely on the point, you could use a small object, a pencil rubber, or the end of a pen or biro. You can even adapt a

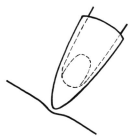

thimble by glueing to its end a small rounded tip of a size which just covers the exact area. The thimble point may also be warmed, to apply heat, but use carefully. This little device may be found very effective, as may other small practical instruments which are available such as electrical vibrators; but the simplest method of all is massage by the tip of the finger.

It should be mentioned that, just as people vary enormously in their sensitivity to medicines, with some requiring up to ten times the dose of certain drugs to get the full effect, so people vary in their response to finger pressure. But, in general, a few minutes should suffice. Similarly, the length of time for which relief lasts will vary from patient to patient, from a few minutes to several hours or even days, but the effectiveness of the point will not vary through use, and the same result will be obtained time and time again.

It is of course usually more difficult to notice a result when the complaint is less painful, but the principle is always the same, however serious the ailment – carry on stimulating the point until you feel relief.

Let us now look at certain common complaints and the tiny pressure points which are the key to relieving them.

Ailments

Aerophagia (air swallowing)

Sufferers from heartburn are familiar enough with this complaint, and yet there is no straightforward medical definition of it. For a long time the excessive belching of aerophagia was thought to be due to a large amount of air in the stomach, but today we know that when we swallow air it doesn't reach the stomach. It only gets as far as the oesophagus, and is then rejected by belching, so with aerophagia we are really talking about a nervous complaint; in fact, it is frequently associated with psychosomatic factors, but often it is acquired as a bad habit, and is due to inability to chew and swallow food properly without also taking in large quantities of air. But belching may also be symptomatic of serious digestive troubles: stomach ulcers, gall stones, and so on, and the stomach distension may also trigger off pain in other areas; for instance pain which is similar to angina.

For these reasons, aerophagia should not be dismissed as unimportant. It is sensible to consult a doctor to find out the specific cause. But in the meantime you will need relief.

For heartburn and distended stomachs, two acupressure points are helpful. Let us look at the first one. Along the inside of the foot, feel the protrusion of the base of the big toe. Put your little finger on this spot and your other fingers alongside as in the photograph below. The end of the index finger will be resting on the first point as it meets the edge of the bone.

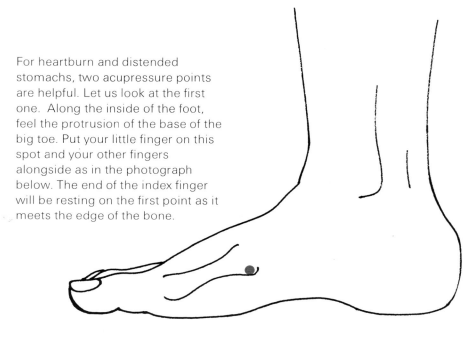

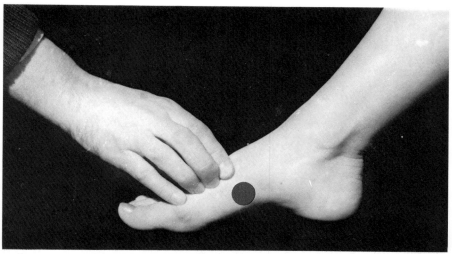

The second point, on the outside edge of the the forearm, may be located in the following way: half bending the arm, the point is halfway along the upper edge between the elbow and the wrist. It will be found about halfway between the skin creases at the wrist and the elbow.

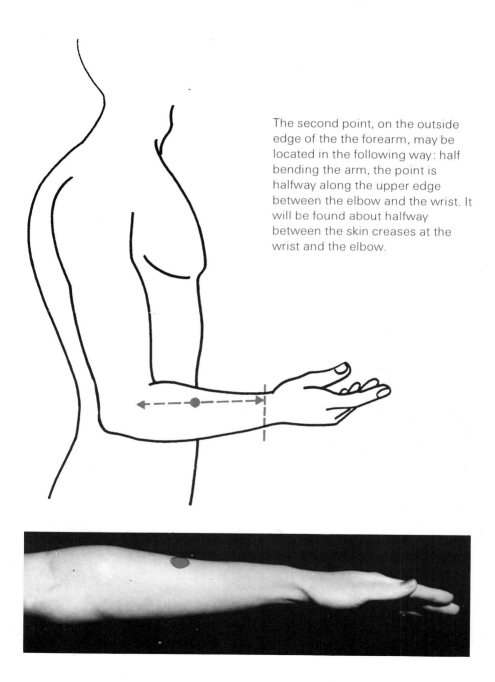

Pains in the anus

Anal pains immediately make us think of haemorrhoids, and in fact this uncomfortable illness is frequently the cause, but you may be suffering for a number of other reasons: anal fissure, the burning and itchiness of eczema, or an infection such as a boil or abscess. Many people suffer from anal pains, and pain from few areas of the body cause such distress and put us in such a bad mood. This is as much due to the pain itself as the physiological malfunction which is associated with it, since the pain inevitably leads to reluctance to open the bowels. Going back to haemorrhoids, the most frequent reason for anal pain, these are varicose veins of the anal region, and although these are not often a sign of a more serious illness, and therefore if they are causing severe or persistent discomfort it is wise to see a doctor, the cause is merely constipation. The passing of infrequent, dry and over-large stools tears these veins, causes swelling, bleeding and blood clots.

These swollen veins cause the anus to shrink and contract, making the passing of stools even more difficult. Thus a vicious circle is set up where pain gives rise to muscle spasms in the anus, and further constipation. So it is important to break the vicious circle as soon as possible by relieving the constipation and establishing regular bowel habits, but when immediate relief of pain is required there is a massage site which is particularly effective.

The point is situated on the back of the calf, halfway up the leg, just in between the swelling of the two prominent calf muscles.

The point corresponds with and is sometimes used for pain in other areas, but it is particularly beneficial for pain in the region of the anus. It should be massaged bilaterally and deeply, and this is most effective if done using both thumbs.

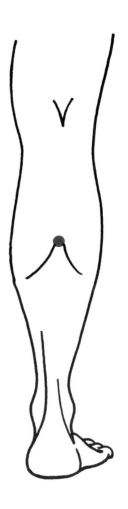

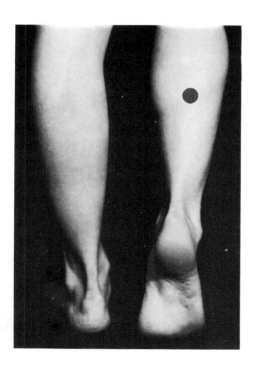

Loss of voice

You have a common cold, and suddenly or gradually your voice changes tone, breaks, or just disappears. Or perhaps you've had to shout excessively at a noisy party, or have given a lecture, and your throat has dried up, and you have lost your voice. This is a nuisance in everyday life, but it is disastrous if you use your voice professionally; the singer loses her quality, the politician loses his voters, and teachers can no longer teach; so we can see how this affliction can have social and professional consequences.

How can we explain this curious disappearance of sound? Our larynx, the organ which produces our voice, contains a pair of 'reeds' which are known technically as the vocal cords. When we speak we cause them to open and close rapidly, and as they move they cause the column of air to vibrate. By constantly modulating this vibration they produce the sounds which come out of our mouths.

Two things may go wrong with our vocal cords. Firstly, they may become inert, and no longer respond to the signals from the nerves, a condition called laryngeal paralysis. This may be serious, and if the loss of voice does not appear to have an obvious cause, such as a cold or sore throat, it is wise to seek the advice of an ear, nose, and throat specialist, so that an accurate diagnosis can be obtained, and immediate treatment started.

Secondly, and fortunately far more frequently, the cause is either excess use, or infection. Inflammation has caused the cords to become swollen so that they cannot move freely and produce proper vibrations. In this instance acupuncture may be very helpful by relieving the congestion of the larynx, and this allows the sufferer to regain his voice.

There are two massage points which are relevant. One is above the wrist. Measure one hand's breadth above the uppermost crease of the wrist, and the point lies on the line that runs up the centre of the forearm and divides it into two halves.

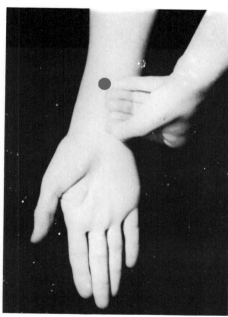

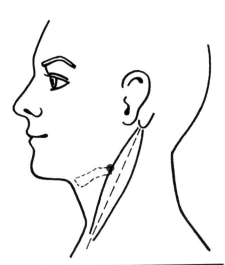

The second is situated on either side of the little bone, called the hyoid, which is above this organ. We see it clearly in the diagram. This point may be massaged gently with the thumb and index finger of the same hand.

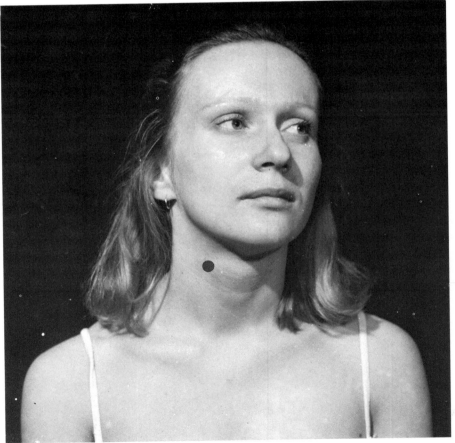

Burns and sunburn

Sunburn, unless very severe, is just one example of a first degree burn. The severity of burns is categorized by degrees. In first degree burns there is redness of the skin; in second degree there are also blisters; a third degree burn involves complete destruction of the whole thickness of the skin, which becomes insensitive, white, or black if carbonized, and completely dead. Fourth and fifth degree burns also exist depending on whether the muscle or bone is affected.

Relatively benign burns, like sunburn, may be helped by finger massage. The extent is important, since even with widespread first degree burns it is wise to see a doctor, and if there are blisters an antiseptic dressing is necessary.

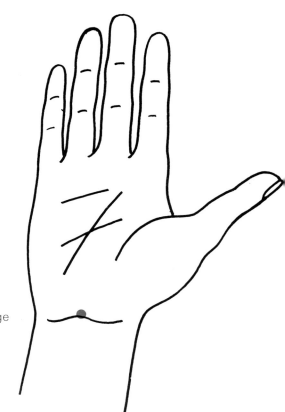

One massage point can relieve burns, whatever their cause. This point is inside the hand, halfway along the fold of the wrist. Massage it strongly, and the burning sensation will diminish considerably.

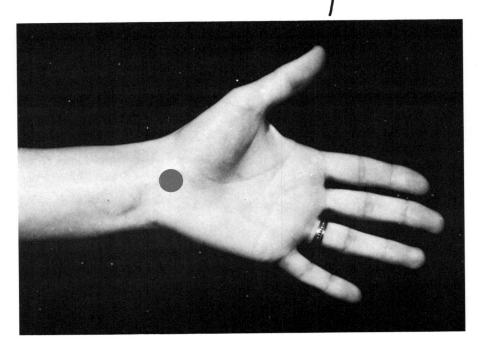

Sprained ankle

This is usually the result of a twisting injury, missing a step, or slipping against the kerb. Such an injury should be taken seriously; you may have a fracture, and you should be X-rayed. But meanwhile, the ankle is swollen and very painful and massage can help.

Apply firm pressure, or massage, to the point situated just below the bottom of the ankle bone, either on the inside or the outside, depending on where the swelling is.

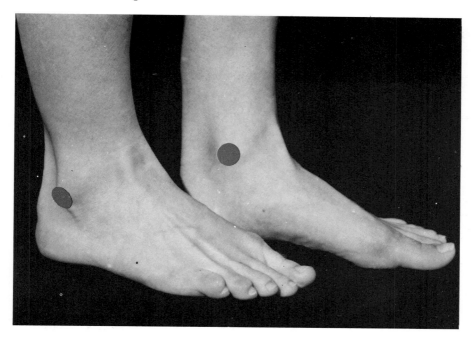

The pain, and even the swelling to some extent, will lessen and you will be able to walk. But again do be careful, massage with the finger perpendicular to the skin simply by pressing, so that you don't displace anything, as this could be unfortunate if there is a fracture, even a partial one; and see your doctor as soon as possible.

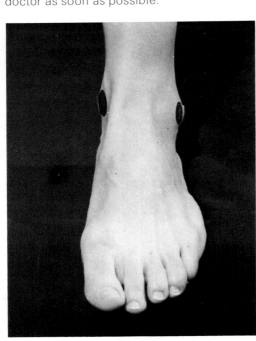

Colic

This word covers a vast range of complaints:

intestinal, affecting either the small or the large intestine. This is the most frequent site, and may be caused by infection, spasms, cold pain etc.

biliary, that is, connected with bile ducts, often caused by a stone.

ureteric, following a urinary infection, or more commonly a stone.

In all these cases, and particularly the last two, the pain can be very sudden and excruciating, sometimes even causing the patient to faint.

Relief is as important as diagnosis, not only because you want to alleviate the pain, but also because further pain merely aggravates the colic. You must try and break this vicious circle, and preferably in a way which avoids use of drugs, since they sometimes make things worse.

The rapid effect of the massage point has been the subject of numerous studies on acupuncture. By recording the rate of intestinal contractions, stimulation is clearly shown to reduce them or to stop them altogether.

This point is situated on the inside of the knee, along the back edge of the tibia.

When we follow this edge with the finger, from bottom to top, we find an angle where the edge of the bone suddenly bends inwards. The point is at this angle.

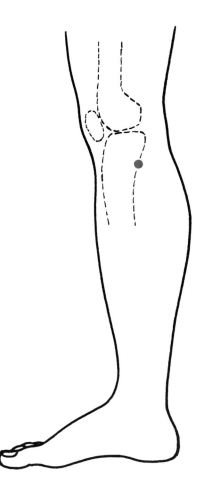

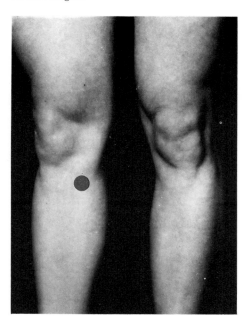

Constipation

This is a common complaint, a disease of the Western world, and of sedentary lifestyles; but it was common in the classical world too, and laxative remedies have even come down to us from the ancient Egyptians.

Nevertheless, there's no doubt that lack of exercise together with an unhealthy diet – not drinking enough liquid, not eating enough roughage, green vegetables, bran and so on – aggravate the problem.

Unfortunately many people resort to taking laxatives, in the form of pills or medicines, and this is merely adding evil to evil. Either the intestine gradually becomes irritated and inflamed, and constipation gives way to diarrhoea which causes dehydration and loss of essential mineral salts; or it becomes habituated to the laxative, and larger and larger doses are required. Thus further complications arise due to laxatives which can lead to chronic complaints and even to serious intestinal diseases. So any natural method which will restore regular bowel movement without traumatizing the body is to be welcomed. Massage is helpful, with one point which is very easy to stimulate.

This point is situated at the inside corner of the nail of the big toe, as in the diagram.

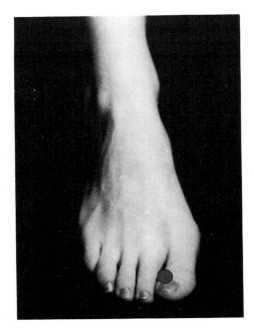

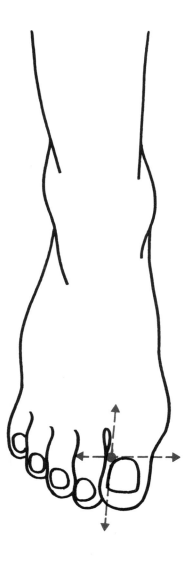

Elbow pain

The elbow is a superficial and an awkward joint, which often gets knocked. And it is also often misused, particularly in sports like tennis and golf. What actually happens? Usually when a shot hasn't quite worked, the forearm goes too far and gets strained. The pain may be felt anywhere in the elbow, but usually on the outside at the lower end of the upper joint bone, the humerus, or 'funny bone'.

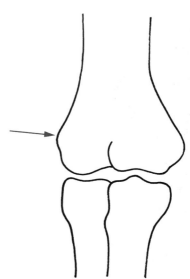

This part of the bone is called the epicondyle, and is attached to a whole complex of muscles, tendons, and ligaments.

When one of these ligaments becomes torn or inflamed, we have what is known as 'tennis elbow'. For a sedentary worker, this may be no more than a nuisance, but for a professional sportsman it can be disastrous for his career. So it is very helpful to know the point which will bring immediate relief and avoid chronic complications.

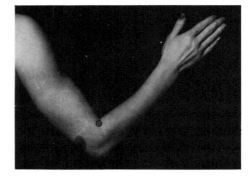

This point is very easy to find. It is at the very inside fold of the elbow when the arm is bent at a right angle.

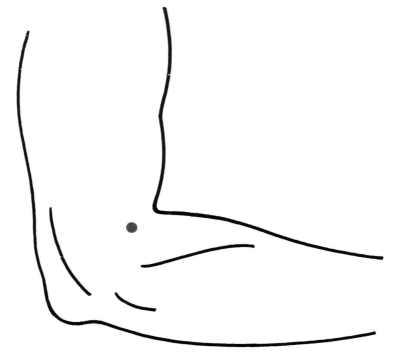

Stimulation of this point may usefully be accompanied by active movements, and can be done during or after physiotherapy.

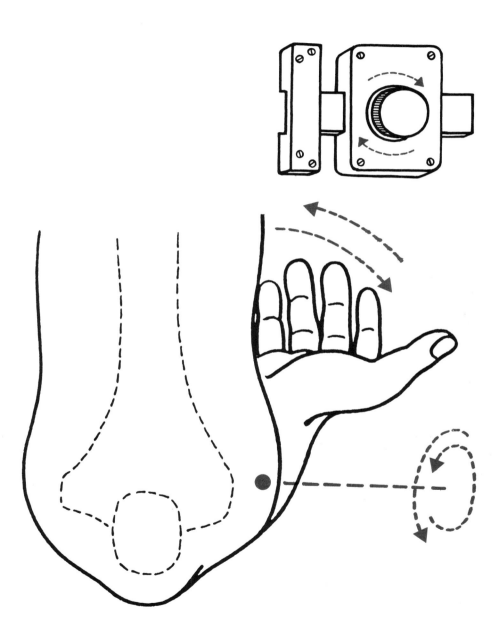

Shock

You must be thinking that this is a strange reason to use acupuncture. When you have had a shock or, to put it scientifically, been traumatized, you usually apply ointment or cream to the affected area, or take an aspirin or a similar analgesic.

This is an interesting point on which to compare the Chinese and Western approaches. In the West, shock is purely and simply seen as the obvious effect of the wound, haematoma (bruise), or fracture, which results in a painful and disturbing sensation. In contrast, for the Chinese this shock is a general effect on the system, disturbing the defence energy which flows throughout the body in a complex network of channels.

So stimulation of a strategic point along one of these channels will improve the patient's condition. It is interesting to note that both the Chinese and Western concepts of shock involve mental and physical trauma; even shock from bad news, or bereavement and mourning.

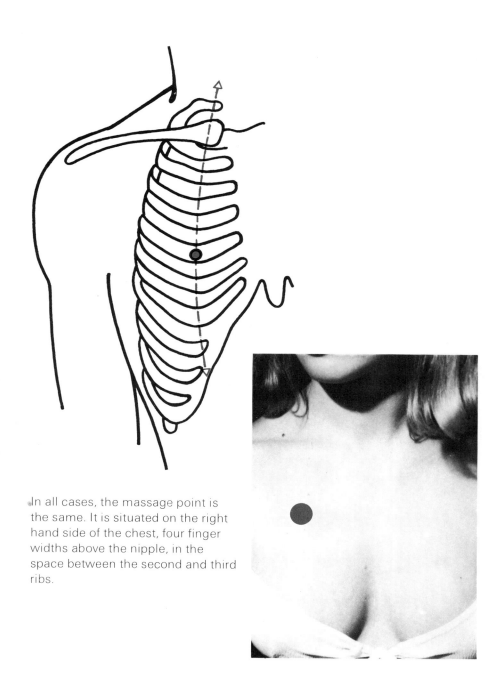

In all cases, the massage point is the same. It is situated on the right hand side of the chest, four finger widths above the nipple, in the space between the second and third ribs.

Leg cramp

Older people, especially, are often woken up in the night by painful muscle cramps. These usually occur in the calf of the leg. There are two sorts of cramps; one is linked to the blood vessels, and is vascular; and the other is linked to malfunctioning of muscles, and is muscular.

Amongst vascular cramps, there are those which often result from varicose veins or phlebitis, and these affect women particularly.

Muscular cramps often follow excessive physical exercise, and occur, for example, in runners, cyclists, and swimmers. There is a point which will bring quick relief from cramps.

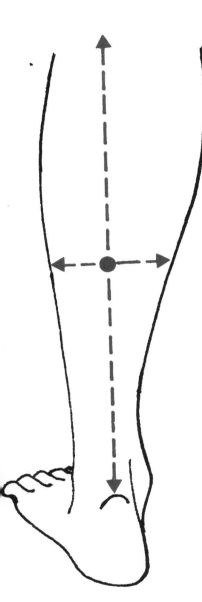

This point is situated on the calf of each leg, right in the middle, halfway round the back and halfway between the bend of the knee and the heel.

More exactly, the point is in the hollow which separates the two large masses of muscle which become prominent when we stand on tip-toe, and are usually the site of the cramp. This is a deep point, for which firm deep massage is recommended.

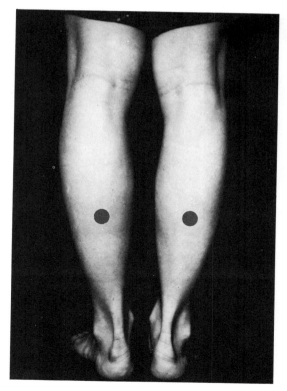

Toothache

Everyone suffers from toothache at some time or another, so it is especially useful to know the effective massage point. Luckily it is easily located.

It is situated on the index finger, on the thumb side, at the point of the right angle formed between the horizontal line of the base of the nail and the vertical line at the side of the nail. Use the point on the index finger of the side where the tooth is aching.

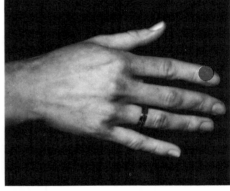

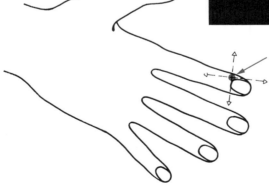

Of course this massage will not cure decay or an abcess, but it will make the delay until you can see a dentist bearable, and it may even help you undergo treatment without anaesthesia. In any case it is worth a try.

Depression

Depression . . . this word is heard only too often today. For no obvious reason, over the course of a few days or weeks, a person previously full of go suddenly loses all interest in life. Work bores him, his family tires him and entertainment is of no interest. A number of physical effects follow; the sensation of being trapped, emotional over-reaction such as shivering, or difficulty in swallowing and a sensation of a lump in the throat, and difficulty in sleeping.

As this usually takes place in a person who is aware of what is happening, his condition disturbs him; he reacts, cries, rebels and revolts against the people who surround him. Alternating phases of excitement and despair are characteristic of depression. Little by little intense fatigue follows the least physical or mental effort. The very idea of moving, of work, of going out, appalls him, his memory deteriorates, and family, social and professional life grinds to a halt. There are numerous physical and psychological causes of depression. Not the least of these is the pressure of everyday life; the tensions and stresses which affect us all, such abnormalities as the air and food pollution which our bodies struggle against, long and exhausting journeys, hectic and demanding work, and the interruption of concentration by telephone calls.

There is a great temptation to resort to drugs and tranquillizers, but the dosage has to be increased before long to obtain the same effect; the senses are deadened and the patient withdraws more and more into his own private world.

Established severe depression is a serious illness which urgently needs medical care. However, it is often possible to prevent it developing if the cause is the external pressure of a stressful and unsuitable way of life.

In such an important state which affects a person in every way, there is no single pressure point, but rather a series of zones which will bring relief.

Lie back comfortably, relax, and
massage the folds of the wrist
which are closest to the palm with
the thumb of the other hand, first in
one direction and then the other.
Then massage the hollow of the
stomach between the navel and the
base of the ribs along the mid-line.

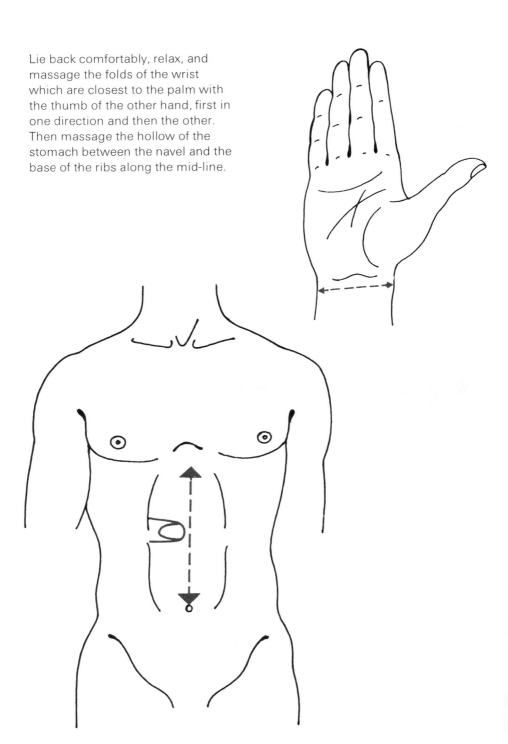

Finally, towards the end of the session, locate the point situated at the highest part of the skull, and massage around it energetically with circular movements. The point will be found along the line joining the ears across the top of the head.

Use this treatment several times a day, and you will gradually notice an improvement which will help you fight the beginning of depression.

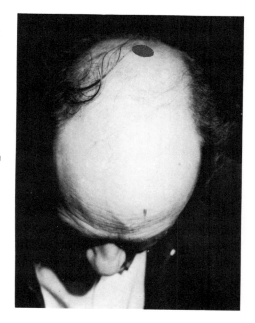

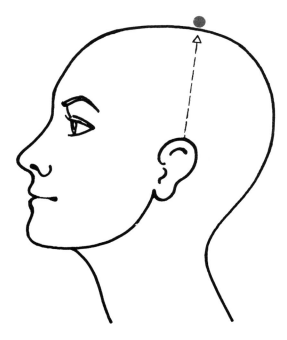

Diarrhoea

Diarrhoea is very unpleasant, and may be caused by one of a number of things. It is serious because it often involves substantial loss of fluid and essential trace elements, thus endangering the body. It may be caused by a simple tummy upset, but it can be more serious if it is due to malabsorbtion or a particularly virulent agent like food poisoning or dysentery, or by a disease which is making a reappearance in tropical countries, even though it was thought to have been almost stamped out — cholera.

Severe diarrhoea needs urgent medical attention, but there is a massage point which is suitable for use in mild cases. I must add that this point is used in China to cure cholera.

This point needs to be located with care; it is a hand's breadth (five finger widths) below the kneecap on the external part of the leg. And it is halfway between the ridges of the tibia and the fibula.

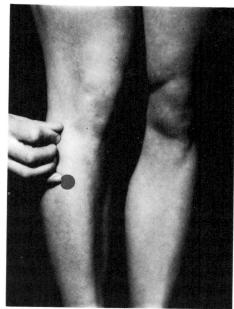

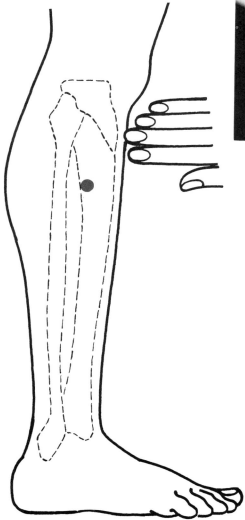

47

Pain in the finger

Fingers are particularly prone to injury. They may be knocked, banged, or strained, or they may be cut, become infected and inflamed.

Everyone is familiar with the way in which the thumbs become painfully deformed in elderly people, due to the development of arthritic conditions.

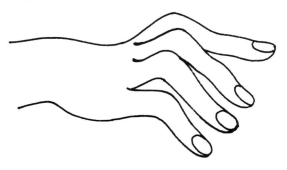

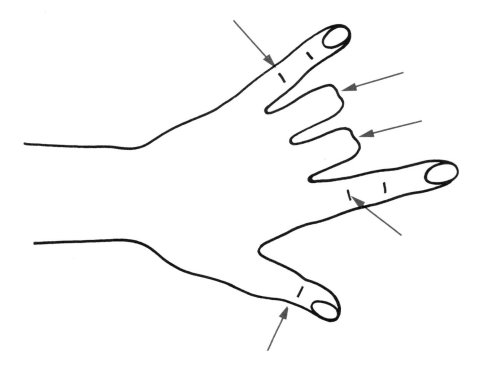

There are massage points which may be helpful. All these points are situated on the back of the fingers, at the bend of the first joint.

Stimulate the point on the affected finger: if all the fingers are affected, Chinese tradition dictates the following order: first the ring finger, then the thumb, the middle finger, the index, and finally the little finger.

Backache

In a society engaged so much in sedentary occupations, the back is inevitably vulnerable. Backache is a familiar enough complaint, and many people do not seem to know the correct way to pick up heavy objects. Such lifting should be done by bending the knees and keeping the back straight; the weight is lifted by straightening the knees, and is taken by the legs and the shoulders, so as to avoid putting a strain on the back. The result of lifting incorrectly, with straight legs and a bent back, is a sudden intense pain; but even worse may be the chronic suffering of typists, pianists, computer operators and dentists. This sort of ache is caused by a persistently bad posture, a curving of the back which causes contractions and spasms of the vertebral muscles. Nor should we forget the aching housewife, who bends to make the bed, to do the washing up, and to do the cleaning and hoovering, day after day!

The back can be affected by many things — uneven pavements, or badly worn heels. The vertebral muscles may even be upset by mental disturbance, by anguish and fear. For example, you arch your back, and may strain it, when confronted with unpleasantness or danger.

All this hurts. So it is useful to know a massage point which will help you relax after the effort, and prevent persistent pain.

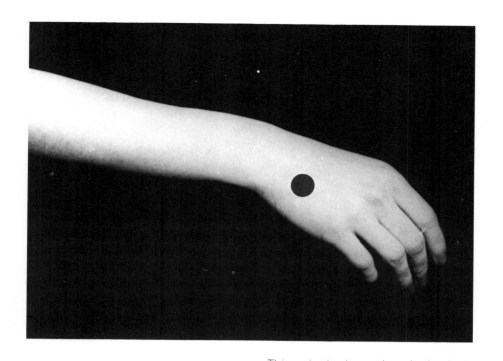

This point is situated on the back of the hand at the angle between the bones which prolong the little finger and the ring finger called fourth and fifth metacarpious.

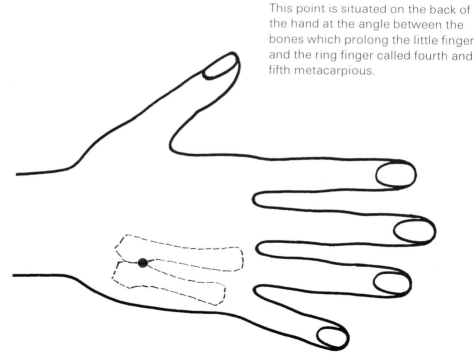

Swelling (oedema)

Oedema can be a sign of a generalized nutritional disease, or of a failure of the heart or the kidneys. In such patients the swelling affects the ankles and feet, unless the person is bedridden, in which case it appears at the bottom of the back. This sort of oedema is a sign of serious illness, and a doctor should be consulted.

But aside from generalized disease, there may be local and less serious causes, such as the oedema caused by varicose veins, particularly common in women, in whom it is often accompanied by phlebitis.

There is also lymphatic oedema, a condition that is likely to be linked to the patient's constitution. This is commoner in women, and produces tree-trunk-like legs.

Also, many people suffer from gravitational oedema, which appears as swelling behind the ankles, and is particularly marked at the end of the day. It occurs particularly in women who have to do a lot of standing or walking, and in those who are on their feet all day, for instance shop assistants or certain types of factory machine workers.

In addition to the appropriate treatment and good advice, such as sufficient rest and sleep, there is a massage point which brings relief.

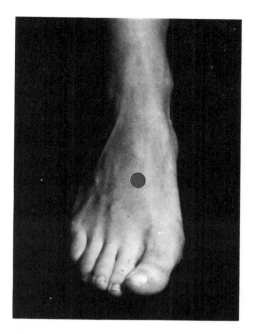

This point is on the foot, at the junction of the bones which prolong the big toe and second toe.

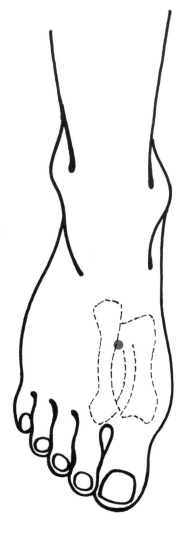

Shoulder ache

The shoulder joint often becomes painful. Sometimes it may be as a result of a direct knock, causing temporary or persistent pain; but more often the pain appears spontaneously, and the most serious effect is that it inhibits activity. The range of movement of the shoulder and arm is restricted, making everyday gestures difficult; doing up a bra, putting on a shirt or jacket, or even driving a car. At the very worst we may suffer from a 'frozen' shoulder, when any movement is almost impossible. This condition may last for only a few days, or up to several months or years. Actually, the joint itself is rarely diseased. The affected parts are the ligaments, muscles, tendons and nerves which surround it, and become damaged and inflamed.

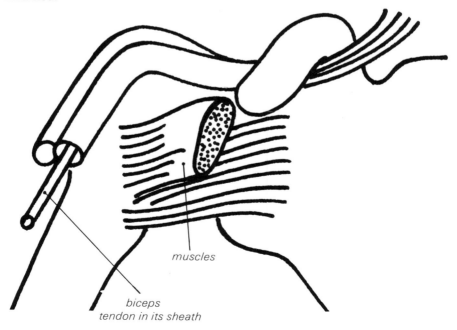

muscles

biceps
tendon in its sheath

The above discussion has outlined the variety of shoulder complaints, but for a general description we may use the term 'periathritis'. Medical methods of treatment include cortisone injections in the shoulder region, and active and passive physiotherapy, including exercise and swimming. But, once again, a point can relieve pain considerably, and prevent the condition from worsening.

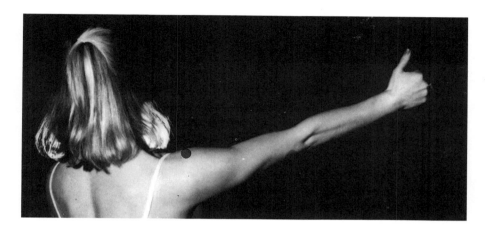

This point is in front of the shoulder, and there is an easy way of finding it. Hold the arm horizontally with the thumb pointing upwards. You'll find a small hollow just in front of the shoulder, and the point is just there. You can also use it during physiotherapy and rehabilitation; it will make your exercises easier. You may also find a number of painful points around the shoulder by pressing. These will vary from one patient to another. Massage them when the need occurs.

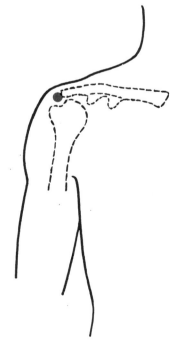

Rash

There are several sorts of rashes. Firstly, those that accompany infectious diseases, such as measles, which are particularly common in childhood. Mostly, apart from chicken pox, these don't itch.

Rashes that do itch, on the other hand, may be of two main sorts. Some are constitutional; they have been with the patient since childhood and often remain throughout life. They demand expert medical care and attention.

Others, however, are fortunately only temporary, and are usually linked to an allergy. Allergies are rather mysterious things. A substance which is totally harmless to the vast majority of people causes the patient to break out in a rash. There are several varieties of these rashes, the most common being eczema, with its dry scales and oozing scabs; but there is also the nettle rash, with its painful, red, velvety swelling which disappears when pressed, and itches dreadfully.

Treatment of an allergy is of course complicated and requires medical advice, but when you break out in a rash from eating strawberries or oysters, for example, it is just as well to be able to relieve the discomfort.

Two massage points are particularly effective. The first is at the back of the knee, exactly half way along the crease of the joint.

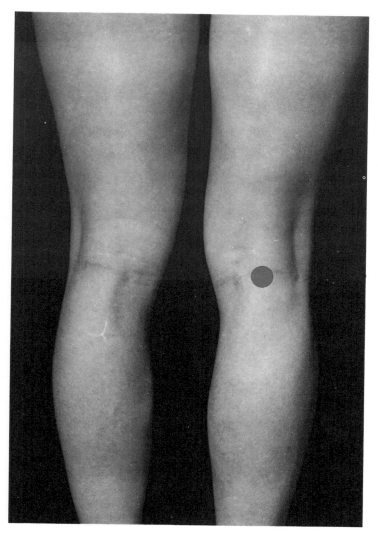

The second is situated on either side of the vertebral column on a level with the third dorsal vertebra. To find it, locate at the base of the nape of the neck a large bony protruberance — this is the spine of the last cervical vertebra. Count three knobs, or spines, below, and you will have reached the third dorsal — our point is on either side, two finger widths along a horizontal line.

To be effective, you need to massage these points quite vigorously.

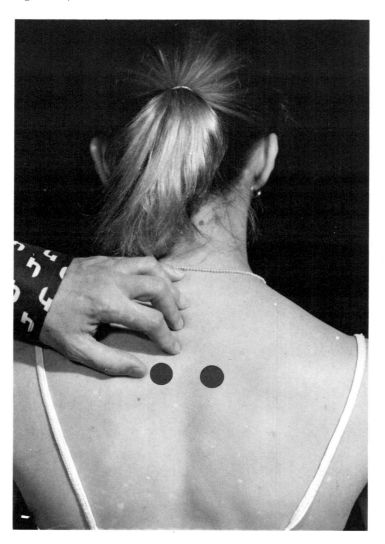

Facial pain

Pains in the face are amongst the least endurable, whether the patient is suffering from facial neuralgia or less easily diagnosed conditions.

Facial neuralgia is a quite specific pain; it is common in older people and occurs quite suddenly after grazing or stimulating a susceptible area on the cheek, the nose or gums. This area is almost always the same for each patient, and is called the trigger zone. The pain is typical; it occurs in a flash, like an electric shock, lasting only a few seconds; but, so the patient tells us, what seconds! The pain is agonizing, and makes the sufferer's life a misery.

In contrast with this quite specific pain, there are several varieties of a different sort of discomfort, where the pain is less intense, but more persistent. Often the face becomes red, and the patient sweats. This is very unpleasant and it is useful to know some points which can bring relief.

There are several points, but two main ones. The first, which is suitable for migraines, headaches, and other facial pains, is situated on the inside of the forearm – use the opposite arm to the side of the pain. Grip with the thumb and index finger round the thumb, and the index will point to the exact spot.

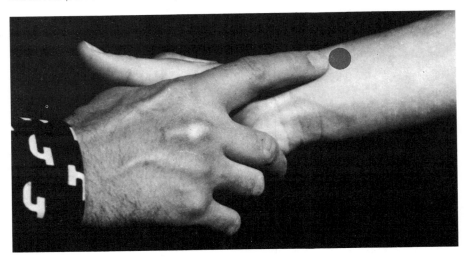

The second point is situated on the
face, level with the nostril in the
bony groove under the cheek.

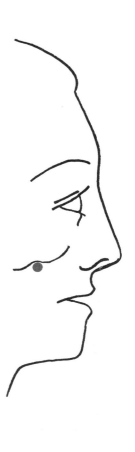

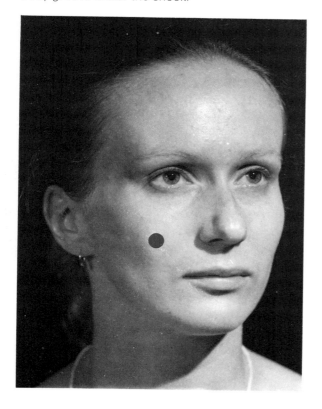

Liverishness

Feeling bilious does not happen, so we are told. Or if it does, it is an inaccurate description of distension of the gall bladder, or of a digestive disturbance, or perhaps it is a polite way to explain the results of overindulgence in food or drink. But the poor man who wakes up with an unpleasant taste in his mouth, a heavy head, a burning sensation in the stomach, and a feeling of nausea that goes on to vomiting, is quite convinced he has a nasty attack!

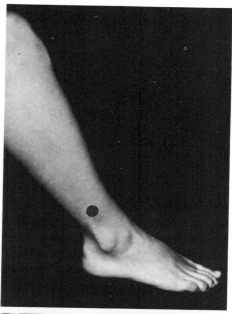

One skin point will relieve you in this situation. It is low down on the outer side of the leg, in a hollow in front of the long thin bone known as the fibula.

How exactly can you find this point? With your fingers together, place your hand on the outside of your leg, with the little finger on the most prominent part of the ankle bone. Your fingers will rest, one above the other, over the fibula and your thumb will mark the spot. Massage this point on both legs with your hands crossed over: right hand for the left leg, and left hand for the right leg. After a while you will hear a gurgling sound in the abdomen. This is the bile emptying, as radiographic examinations which have been taken during the course of the treatment have shown.

Note that this is a very important point for the treatment of all liver and biliary complaints.

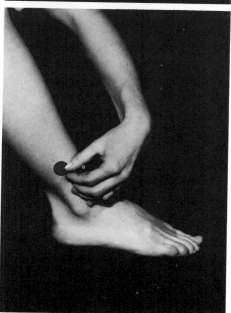

Breathlessness

Technically we call this symptom, which may be a sign of serious illness, dyspnea. Affections of the heart, the lungs, or the nervous system may be the cause. So if you should develop this symptom for no apparent reason, you should see your doctor, and perhaps even a heart or chest specialist. But breathlessness may be only a temporary problem arising from a nasty bout of flu or bronchitis, or even emotion. There is also increasing evidence, as a result of research in California and at the London Hospital, that neurological mechanisms and reflexes may be involved, and these, of course, are susceptible to acupuncture.

One disease in particular is characterized by difficulty in breathing, especially breathing out, and that is asthma. Most people are familiar with its development. In many cases it may be brought on by exposure to something, such as pollen, to which the person is sensitive. In older people it is associated with heart trouble, and causes the patient to wake up at two or three o'clock in the morning, unable to breathe, forcing him to sit in front of an open window. Gradually the attacks become more frequent, and develop into a permanent difficulty in breathing.

Asthma is an unpleasant illness for the patient, and is very distressing for bystanders, who feel helpless. There are a number of medicines which may relieve the asthmatic patient of his breathlessness; usually they contain a sort of cortisone, in the form of drops, pills or aerosol sprays, often combined with drugs to dilate the air passages. But all of these medicines have their disadvantages. Firstly you need to have them at hand; and secondly, all of them have considerable side effects, and can even be dangerous if taken in excess. So it is useful to know a method which can bring rapid relief to the breathless sufferer.

There is a bilateral massage point situated on the back, on either side of the spine and two finger widths away from the centre, at the level of the third dorsal vertebra. To find this vertebra, the patient should sit down and lower his head. You will notice a projection at the base of his neck, which is the projection of the last cervical vertebra. Going down the back, count three more protrusions, and you will have reached the level of the third dorsal. The point is situated at two finger widths on the left and right of the spine. The point needs to be massaged energetically for a considerable time — so the patient will need help from someone. Gradually the breathlessness and wheezing will ease until the difficulty disappears, but if the attack is very severe, medical help should be obtained urgently.

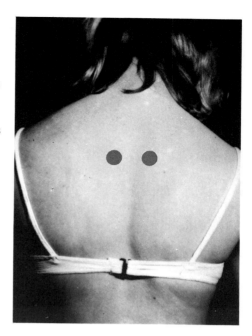

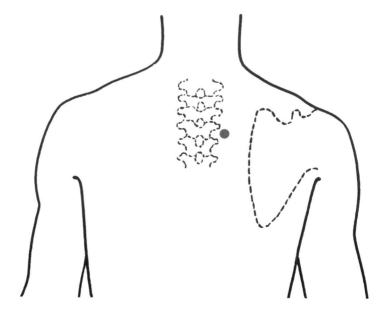

Pain in the knee

The knee joint is vulnerable to bumps, accidents and infections. It is frequently injured in car and sports accidents, and is also highly sensitive to a degenerative change in old age, osteoarthritis, which may become very painful. Getting relief is therefore a frequent problem.

In nature, good and evil often go side by side: thus, although the knee joint is a relatively exposed joint, unprotected by thick muscle masses, the very fact that it is just under the skin makes it very easy to examine and to locate the injured sites.

Besides, and this is valuable for acupuncture as a whole — even when we do not say so directly — a painful point can always be massaged, and this can be as effective as using a specific massage point, and even more so if combined with it. But there is a specific point for the knee.

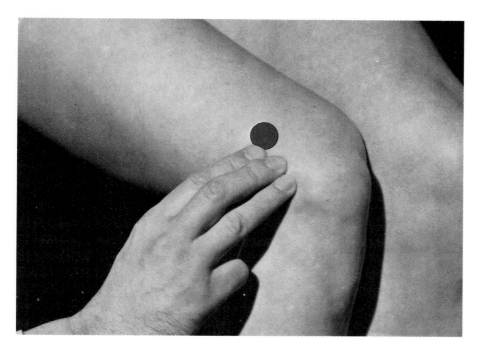

This point corresponds in position with the highest point of the synovial membrane — the little sac which lines the inside of the joint, and which, when the joint is injured or inflamed, swells with inflammatory or haemorragic fluid, a synovial effusion.

How can you locate the point? It is easy. Find the patella, the knee cap, which is the small bone situated in front of the knee. Our point is three fingers widths above the top of the patella, on the outer side of the thigh, as shown in the illustration.

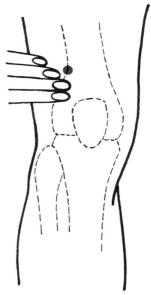

Sore throat

Care is necessary here, since a sore throat may be very serious. It can signal the beginning of several other diseases – meningitis, rheumatic fever or kidney disease – which can have a lasting effect on your life, so unless the sore throat is mild, see your doctor quickly. But meanwhile there is a point which will bring relief.

This point is situated on the side of the thumb facing the index finger. Draw a line along the base of the nail – draw a second line at right angles along the side of the nail. The point is at the right angle formed by these two lines. If you have a sore throat on one side only, massage the point on this side only. If you have a sore throat all over, massage both sides energetically, either alternating or simultaneously.

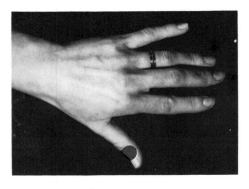

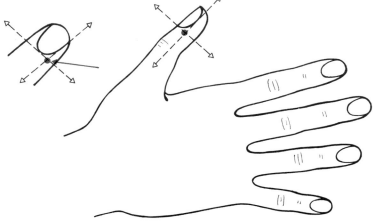

Influenza

The symptoms are familiar enough: you catch a chill, and soon you have watery eyes, a burning sore throat, a running nose, and you sneeze and feel shivery ... and you rush for a hot whisky or brandy — which has never done any good: alcohol only kills germs if it is applied to them directly with cotton wool!

We say we have got influenza, but this is generally inaccurate. Real influenza is a major disease which comes in epidemics and in its most serious form it can kill, in spite of all the advances of modern medicine.

Usually what has happened when we think we've got flu is that the lining of our air passages, in other words our respiratory mucous membranes, are attacked by one of any number of viruses that are going around, and which give us a cough, a runny nose, and a temperature. This means we have got a cold. It is striking how well popular wisdom compares with the Chinese concept of cold as an unsympathetic energy which invades the body, and comes up against the 'guard dogs', a select set of the acupuncture meridians. This, according to Chinese theory, is a complex mechanism which we can only mention here, but there are some major points that should be stimulated, and these lie along these meridians. When one feels the onset of a cold, the two main points should be stimulated, as soon as possible.

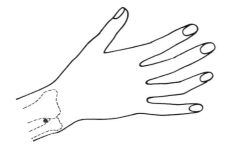

The first point is on the back of the wrist, three finger widths above the crease.

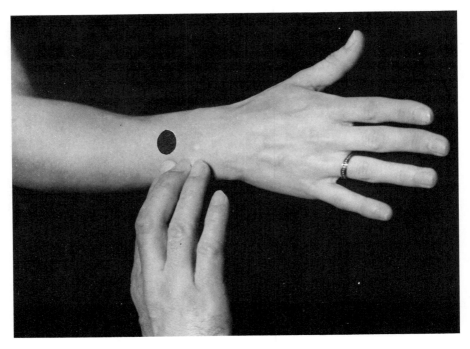

The second point is situated on the
slope of the shoulder halfway
between the base of the neck and
the shoulder tip.

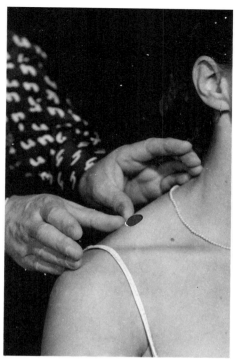

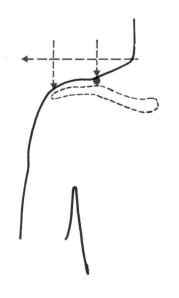

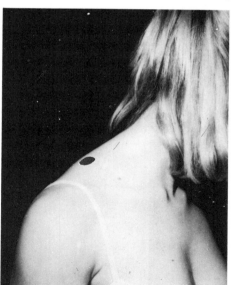

Pain in the hip joint

One thing should be mentioned straightaway. An ache in the hip need not be due to an affection in the hip joint itself. It may also be a sign of infection in the abdomen, or of trouble in the lower part of the back. This is because the same set of nerves is involved. In such cases, the point recommended below will not be of much use, since it is only concerned with conditions in the hip joint itself.

The hip is a deep joint, and is generally well protected by ligaments and muscles, but as it bears the whole weight of the body, it tends to be affected by osteoarthritis, a slow and dreadfully destructive disease which eventually, after much pain and restriction of movement, causes the joint to become fixed in one position.

There have been some brilliant advances in the methods of treating osteoarthritis, and nowadays surgeons can replace the whole hip joint with a metal or plastic one.

However, there is a useful massage point which can relieve pain and help associated treatment, such as exercise, heat, or physiotherapy. You should locate it carefully.

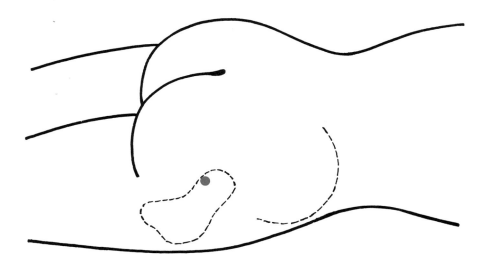

The patient should lie on his healthy side and half bend his affected leg. This position allows the bones to stand out in relief — in particular the protrusion of the pelvis and the iliac crest.

Place your hand along the crest in the following manner: open your hand with the fingers straight and together, and with your thumb at right angles to them; place the heel of your hand along the crest, with the thumb pointing forwards. The tip of your middle finger will then be on the point — in anatomical terms, it is on the bony prominence known as the 'greater trochanter', as in the diagram, which you can feel under the skin.

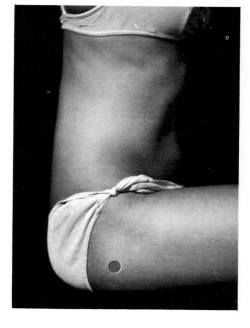

Massage of this point even has an effect on all the aches of the lower limb. This is another example of a point which is relevant to more than one complaint.

Hiccups

We all get hiccups occasionally, and they may be embarrassing, or if prolonged and severe, an unpleasant nuisance. But it is not generally known that there can be dreadfully prolonged attacks which may last days, producing real disability that prevents the sufferer from eating, drinking, and sleeping, and bringing him to the brink of a nervous breakdown. Hiccups usually occur if you have swallowed and something has gone down 'the wrong way', or laughed a great deal, maybe whilst eating. Hiccups are actually caused by sudden contractions, twitching, or spasms of the diaphragm, the thin sheet of muscle which goes across the inside of the body, is attached to the lower ribs, and separates the chest from the abdomen. It is one of the muscles of respiration, and normally it rises and falls smoothly. When it twitches, however, it jerks the ribs, the contents of the chest, and the windpipe, downwards, and that is actually what is happening when we have hiccups.

Usually the cause of hiccups is quite trivial, but it can sometimes be a symptom of serious nervous disease, or chronic kidney failure. But leaving the more serious causes aside, it is desirable to be able to relieve ourselves quickly of the familiar and unpleasant symptoms of a bout of hiccups. To do this, you will need help, since the massage points are on the back. This makes sense, since they are near the very points where the diaphragm is attached to the ribs.

These points are on either side of
the spinal cord at a distance of two
finger widths from the mid line, on a
level with the seventh dorsal
vertebra.

The subject should be seated and
stripped to the waist. The points are
on the horizontal line joining the
lower tips of the shoulder blades, as
shown below.

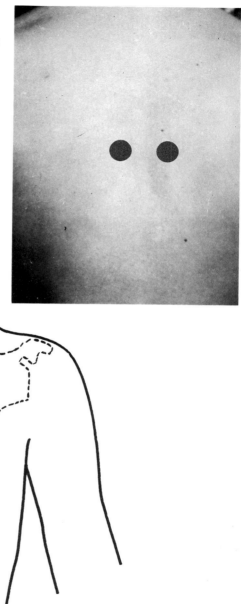

Insomnia

You toss and turn in bed ... the very bed you've been looking forward to throughout a long and tiring day at work. Your nerves are getting the better of you, and you cannot get to sleep. Or you may come home exhausted, sleep like a log until two o'clock in the morning, and then find yourself wide awake. Your mind is full of worries that plague you until the alarm goes off, cruelly announcing that it is time to get up, just as you were beginning to doze off. This is quite serious, since continued tiredness and lack of sleep may lead to depression.

So what should you do? Take a sleeping pill? Thousands are bought every day, but it is not the right solution. It has been discovered — only relatively recently — that sleep is not the simple process that we have always thought. It is a more complex state, with two levels of unconsciousness which alternate and follow on from each other during the course of the night. One level is heavy sleep, when the body, and especially the eyeballs, are still, and this sleep rests the body: the other level is paradoxical sleep, where the brain is very active and the eyeballs move about, so called 'Rapid Eye Movement' or REM sleep. It is during REM sleep that you dream, and it has been found, by waking up volunteers doing experiments on sleep, that dreaming is essential for mental health. REM sleep is also the time when your mind resolves the problems that have been troubling you during the day. Now, no sleeping pill can act without disturbing this delicate balance; almost all have been found to produce only deep sleep, leaving a 'hangover' next morning. The insomnia inexorably becomes chronic, and the sufferer has to increase the dosage of sleeping pill, adding one drug to another, while his health gradually breaks down. So, any natural method which can help you to sleep is more than welcome.

There are two points which will help, and you should massage them slowly. The first one is situated at the end of the second toe — the one next to the big toe; and the point is at the outer angle of the nail.

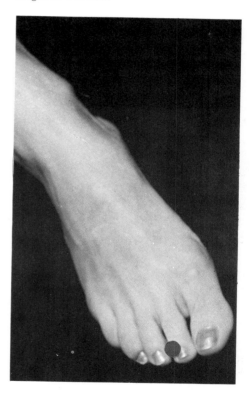

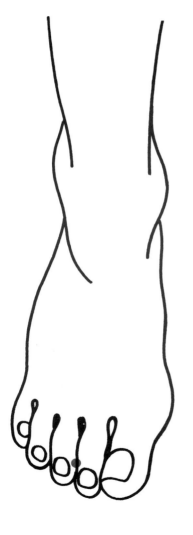

The second point is situated on the inside edge of the foot along the side of the big toe, and behind the bony protrusion of the base of the big toe.

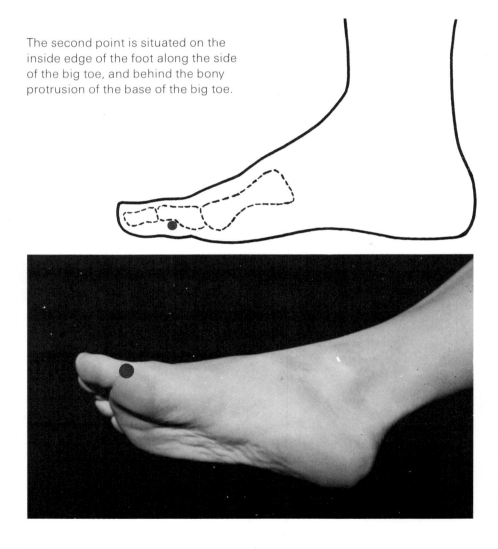

Intoxication

The Chinese faced the problem of drug addiction long before the West was aware even of its existence, let alone its gravity. It is not surprising, then, that they were able to discover an effective acupuncture point for treatment of addiction to opium and its derivatives; this point is still valid and brings results which are equally successful in the West. What is more, it has been found to be fruitful also in the treatment of alcohol and tobacco addiction, if used in combination with one or two other select points. Partial or total cure of addiction is of course of great importance and interest to us.

Drugs

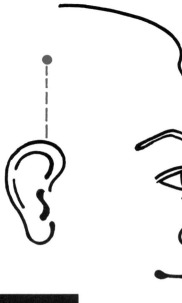

The major point for all addiction is the *drug* point. This is situated on the side of the skull exactly in line with the highest point of the ear, and three finger widths above it.

This point is effective for hard or soft drugs: opium, LSD, hashish, addiction to sleeping pills and so on.

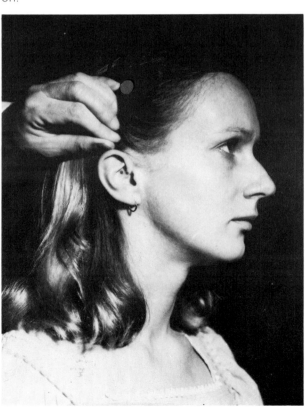

Alcoholism

When drunkenness is common, an additional point is important. It is situated exactly at the tip of the nose, and is called the P-Tchoun; massage here will have a rapidly sobering effect. But take care: stimulation of this point can cause vomiting. Stand at the patient's side, and not right in front of him!

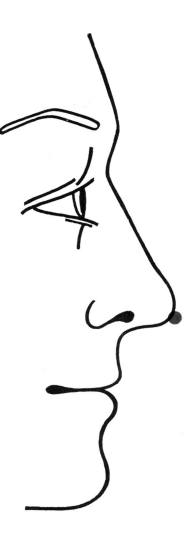

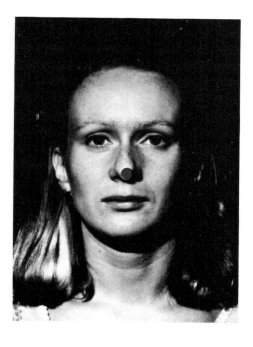

Tobacco

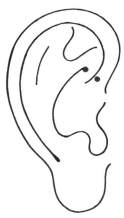

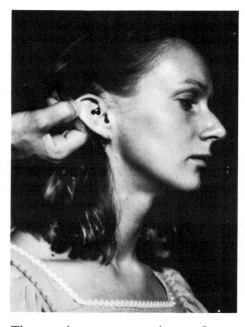

The major *drug* point, as mentioned before, should be stimulated. Two other points on the ear are also effective. One of them is situated on the tiny bridge of flesh which forms the 'root' of the ear and is called the root or 'helix'.

The second point is just behind it, almost in the middle of the hole formed by the outer shell of the ear, which is so similar to the inside of an oyster that it has been called the conch.

These points occupy a tiny surface area, and it is not easy to find them; but, once located, it is sufficient to massage these points several times a day, and addiction to tobacco will lessen.

These points allow us to mention an interesting extension of classical acupuncture. French researchers, in particular, Dr Nogier, and a number of Chinese, have studied an area which until now had escaped the attention of traditional investigation. This is the outer part of the ear, and an entire science has arisen out of it – 'auriculotherapy'.

So we can see that the age of discovery in acupuncture is not over, and there may still remain other points and useful techniques yet to be revealed.

Tired legs

City-dwellers lead a shamefully sedentary existence all week. We sit all day at the office or in the car, then we try to get a week's exercise all on one day. Off we go on Sunday for a walk, a ramble, or for more violent sports, and it doesn't take long for us to get tired ... we can't feel our legs, or rather we can feel them aching only too well!

You need not go so far! But if you sit down and massage it for a long time, you will feel that the tiredness in your legs has disappeared.

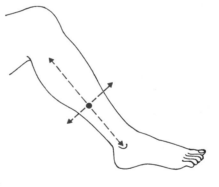

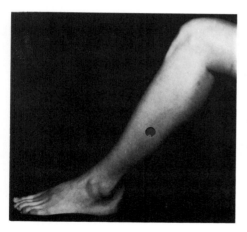

There is a point that is effective in relieving our fatigue. It is on the outer side of the leg, halfway between the ankle and the knee, just behind the long thin bone known as the fibula.

The point was known in China as the 'coolies point' after the indefatigable men who used to carry heavy loads for days on end without tiring. During the last war, the Japanese soldiers, who covered vast distances on foot or by bicycle in the jungle, would burn this point with a lighted cigarette end every twenty kilometres, and carry on again, quite refreshed.

Lumbago

All of us have suffered from lumbago, or backache, at some time or another. It usually occurs after we have over exerted ourselves with the back in an awkward position. In just a second the back goes . . . and we are doubled up, and often incapable of getting up, since the very least movement is excruciatingly painful. Sometimes the cause is a slipped disc, and sometimes the pain is due to a displaced vertebra. Whichever it may be, the nerve is caught and pressed on, the muscles contract into spasm, and we feel intense pain. Usually, however, the cause is more trivial, a slight tear in a ligament or muscle, caused by a sudden twist or strain.

If lumbago isn't treated it may drag on for several days or weeks, improving very slowly, and only gradually will it eventually disappear. And you may suffer a relapse, unless you are careful, and at increasingly regular intervals – as the ligaments, which hold the vertebrae together, become strained; and you will get these attacks after less and less strenuous exertion. Soon you will have a constant ache, with recrudescences following tiredness, and on getting up in the morning. You have become a chronic sufferer from lumbago.

There is a massage point which will relieve lumbago, and it is very easy to find. It is exactly in the middle of the fold of the knee at the back of the leg. This point may be used on both legs.

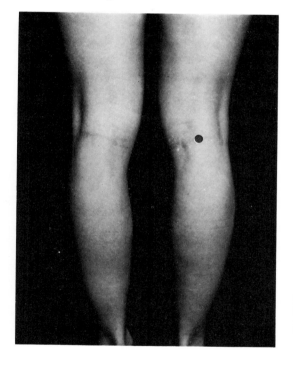

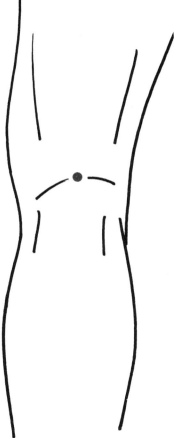

Ache in the wrist or hand

It is virtually impossible to separate aches in the wrist from aches in the hand. There is a whole network of bones, tendons and muscles which link the two, as shown in the diagram below.

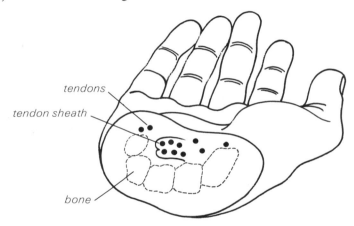

Sometimes a swelling, not always painful, appears on the back of the hand or the wrist; this is a synovial cyst. The fine membrane which lines the joints between the different bones in the wrist, and also lubricates the tendons, the 'synovial' membrane, herniates through the ligaments, and forms a small swelling under the skin. It is filled with a thick, viscous fluid, like treacle. This happens after a violent movement has damaged the ligament, often in tennis players, or when straining with a screwdriver: it may also occur after frequently repeated movements, as in basket making and weaving.

Also, sometimes the ligamentous band across the front of the wrist, which holds the tendons in place, becomes inflamed or shrinks, and compresses the nerves which run underneath it. This will produce a neuralgic pain in the wrist or the hand, and signs of swelling may appear around the wrist or the palm.

For all wrist and hand pains, two acupuncture points are particularly helpful.

The first is on the little finger side of the hand, a little beyond the wrist, on the second fold which forms when the hand is bent forward as shown in the photo and explained in the diagram.

The second point is situated on the back of the wrist, three finger widths above the fold just where the two bones of the forearm meet, the radius and the ulna. This point is very easy to find and feel.

These are the two points to stimulate to relieve a pain in the wrist or hand; they may be used either successively or simultaneously, for as long as is necessary to produce relief.

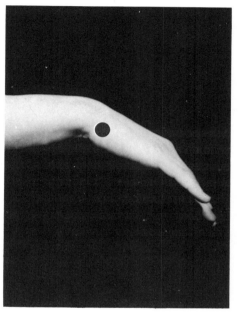

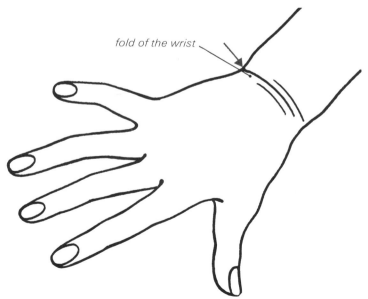

fold of the wrist

Travel sickness

Travel sickness can occur whatever the method of transport – train, car, plane, coach or boat. It starts with a giddy feeling, then nausea and cold sweats develop, finally there is a feeling of sickness, and vomiting. Sometimes you may be on the point of fainting, and this prevents you from eating as you normally would, and keeping up your strength. It can ruin your journey, and people who are prone to travel sickness get to the state where they are afraid to travel. In little children, especially, repeated vomiting can cause dangerous dehydration. It is useful, therefore, to know of an effective point to help on these unpleasant occasions.

The point is situated on the front of the abdomen, right in the middle between the navel and the small point at the bottom of the breast bone in the front of the chest, the sternum.

The point is half way between these two anatomical landmarks, and should be massaged strongly for a long time.

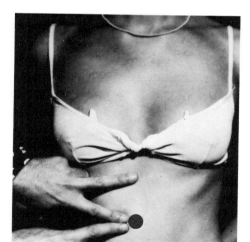

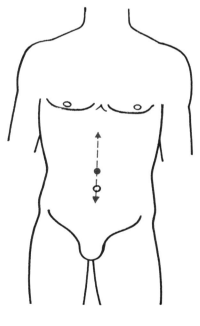

Blocked nose

Unless it is due to hay fever, this is very much a winter ailment. A blocked nose is often the first sign of one of any number of possible virus infections which are common at this time of year: colds, flu and so on.

There are also a series of chronic infections; the nose and related anatomical cavities may be the cause. These include infections of the sinuses, and the spasmodic coryza whose springtime form resembles hay fever, with its sneezing bouts, continually running nose, and soreness and irritation of the eyes.

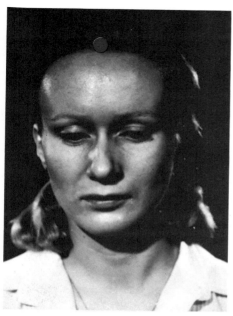

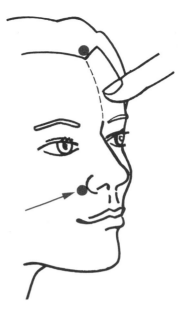

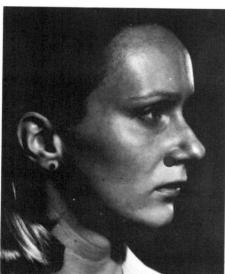

The massage points are the same for all complaints. There are two. One of these is essential and is situated in the middle of the forehead above the hairline; if there is no hair it is even easier to find. Run your finger centrally up the forehead from the bridge of the nose until you reach a small bump, and you'll find the hollow just beyond it; in most people it is just beyond the hairline. Apply firm massage to this spot.

In addition, you can also stimulate the following additional points, which are useful. If one nostril is more congested than the other, there is a point at the bottom corner of the nostril: massage the right side for the right nostril and the left for the left nostril.

Earache

Surprising though it may sound, there are really three ears, or, at least, three parts, not one, which follow upon each other; the external ear, that is, the outer shell and the auditory canal which leads to the drum; the middle ear, a resonating cavity with four linked small bones which transmit the sound; and the inner ear, which registers the sounds, and, amongst other things, contains the mechanism which allows us to keep our balance. This inner ear does not give us pain – disturbance of it is manifested in other ways, such as dizziness, ringing in the ears, deafness, and so on, and we are not concerned with that here.

In contrast, the other two parts of the ear may become painful. Small boils can occur on the outer ear, and are very painful. More seriously, there can be infection in the middle ear which becomes the seat of what is medically known as otitis, and used to be a common cause of deafness, before we had antibiotics.

Otitus is extremely painful and may lead to complications, particularly in the neighbouring bone, the mastoid. Complications usually mean partial loss of hearing, which may affect the patient for the rest of his life. Small children are particularly vulnerable to ear infection, and may need to have an incision made in the eardrum under anaesthetic, to let the pus out.

An ear acupuncturist – such specialists do exist – would be very satisfied to see the patient's ear ooze with pus while it is being stimulated, so as to avoid surgery.

There is a massage point which will relieve simple earache. It is situated just behind the ear, on the mastoid bone. Pull the ear forward and the point is just on the bone.

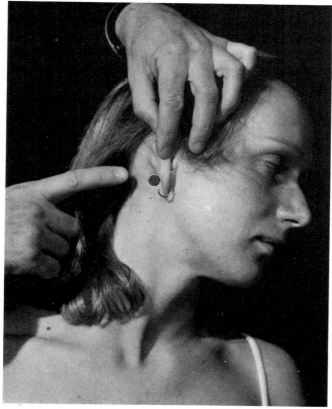

Palpitations

Are we really aware of the astonishing electrical machinery that makes up our hearts, with its own power station and distribution network which stimulates the cardiac muscle to contract regularly? This power station, known medically as the 'pacemaker', normally discharges an electrical signal into the heart about seventy times a minute, and it adapts instantaneously to the needs of the body, depending on whether we are at rest, walking or running, and so on. So complex a machinery may of course go wrong from time to time; a power station may accelerate, or slow down, conditions known to doctors as tachycardia or bradycardia; or it can cause an irregular beat outside of the normal rhythm – which is called an extra-systole.

The recognition, diagnosis, interpretation and treatment of these anomalies require detailed cardiographic investigation, and fortunately the condition is often not serious. As a rule the complaint is recognized by the patient himself. The symptom is one or several palpitations, that is, a sensation of an irregularity, a sudden beat and a pause, or a fluttering sensation in the chest. For a few moments there is a feeling of great anxiety; and the palpitations may be repeated, they may continue for hours, and even become an almost permanent disability. Even if occasional, they can be extremely unpleasant, so it is helpful to try to relieve the patient of them as soon as possible.

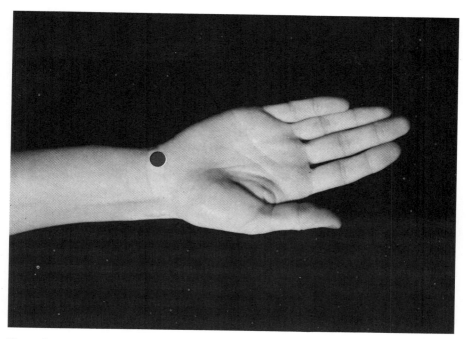

There is one point which is very effective. This point is on the inside of the wrist (that is, on the little finger side), and at the level of the skin fold along the wrist joint.

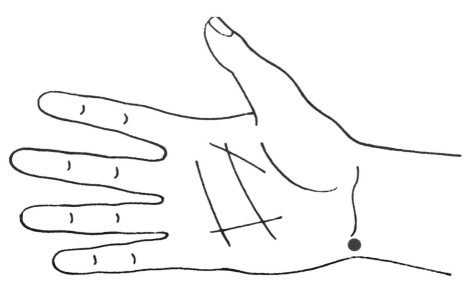

Pain in the foot and toes

Our poor feet suffer throughout the year. They may be cramped inside ill-fitting shoes, or perched up and distorted by stiletto heels or platform soles. In ten years' time you will find yourself with deformed feet, your toes crowded one over the other, and your arch fallen; corns and bunions appear where the foot has been rubbed, walking becomes a torture, and gradually you are forced to seek relief by a surgical operation. The Chinese have been faced with this problem for a long time; their tradition forced the young girls to have their feet bound tightly to keep them small. Inevitably this was painful, and an effective point has been used for a long time to bring relief.

This point is situated on the foot, exactly at the base of the second toe. Stimulate it forcefully to soothe the pain.

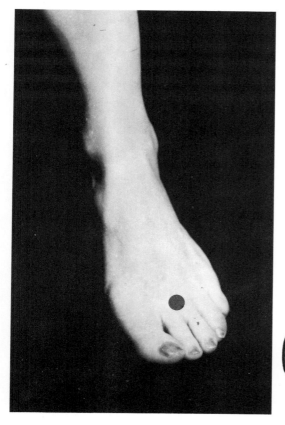

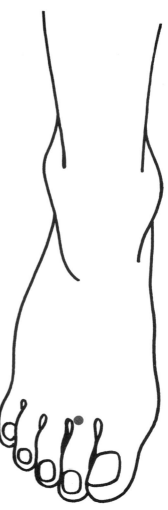

Chest pain

Pain in the chest may originate in the organs inside it, the heart and the lungs, or in the chest wall, the muscles, nerves and ribs. If pain appears without any obvious reason, such as injury, it is wise to take it seriously to start with, and you should arrange to see your doctor, as you may have trouble with your heart or lungs, especially if the onset is sudden. Everyone has heard of coronary thrombosis (heart attack) but chest pains may also be a sign of angina, in which case they come on after exertion. A pulmonary embolus (clot on the lung), is another cause of acute severe chest pain.

However, pains in the chest usually spring from very minor causes, and often the severity of the pain is out of all proportion to the seriousness of the cause. One type of pain that we all know is the 'stitch'. Another is intercostal neuralgia, which may originate near the vertebra; and also, the chest is the most frequent site for the eruption of the infectious and very painful virus disease which has the medical name *herpes zoster*, but is commonly called shingles. Meanwhile, you will need relief.

The massage point is right in the middle of the back of the arm, exactly halfway between the elbow and the wrist. Massage it strongly. Using acupuncture in this point alone, Chinese surgeons have removed parts of the lung without any other form of anaesthesia.

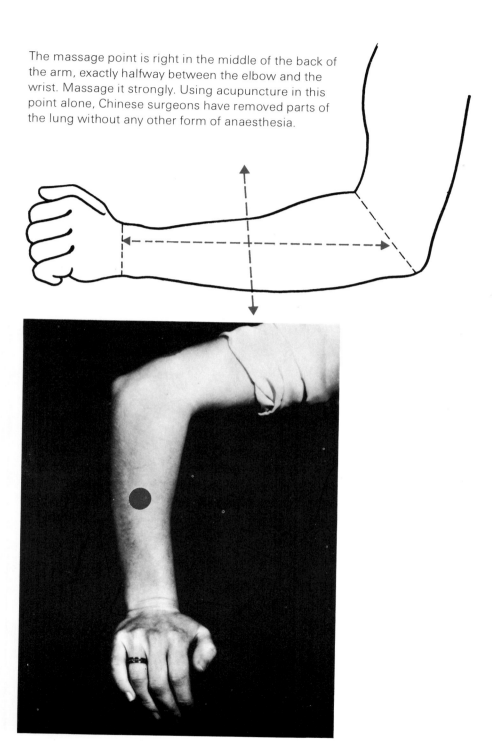

Heavy periods

You may bleed between periods, metrorrhagia, or have periods which are too long or too heavy, menorrhagia. Although many women seem to put up with these complaints remarkably well, vaginal hemorrhage should be attended to without delay as a considerable amount of blood may be lost, and if this occurs regularly, severe anaemia will result. The apparent quantity lost is often not a sign of the real seriousness of the condition; a reduction in blood loss after heavy periods may be a sign of anaemia. So excessive bleeding should be attended to as soon as possible to avoid complications, and a doctor should be consulted without delay.

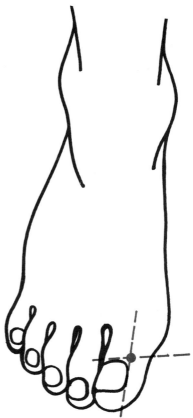

In the meantime, there is an effective pressure point on the foot, in the right angle between the base of the big toe and the outer side of the nail, as shown in the diagram.

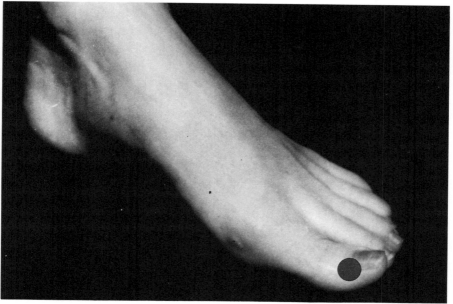

Painful periods

Most women suffer varying degrees of discomfort during their period, whether it be merely a nagging ache, or a violent pain which may even be so agonizing and acute as to cause loss of consciousness from fainting. Although this is a temporary disability, it occurs regularly and predictably, and is awaited with resignation or dread, depending on the severity of the symptoms. And these, and the accompanying psychological disturbance, often have social and professional consequences. Research has shown that women are more likely to be involved in domestic mishaps and even in more serious things, such as car accidents, around the time of their period.

So for the student who has an 'off day' and so fails an exam, or for any woman who feels so indisposed as to be forced to stay away from work, or to cancel her engagements for the day, painful periods are no joke. We need a means of providing fast relief, and there is one point which is very effective for all gynaecological upsets.

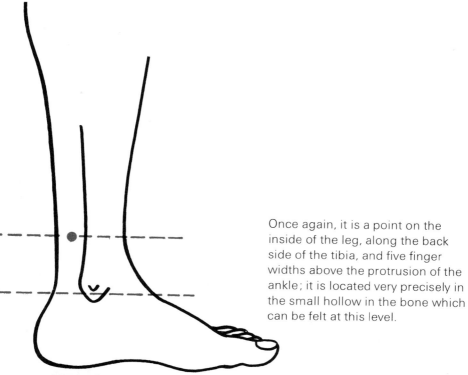

Once again, it is a point on the inside of the leg, along the back side of the tibia, and five finger widths above the protrusion of the ankle; it is located very precisely in the small hollow in the bone which can be felt at this level.

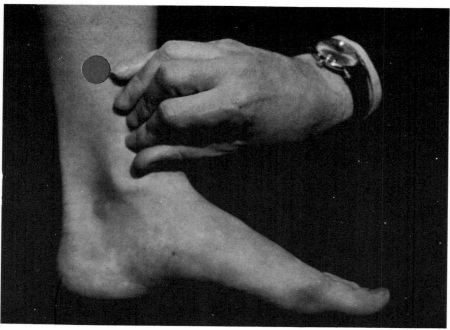

Sciatica

This is one of the more painful complaints from which human beings may suffer. As the name suggests, the complaint centres around the sciatic nerve. This nerve begins with several roots at the level of the lumbar vertebrae column, and these roots gather into one trunk, which passes down the buttock, the back of the thigh and the leg, and ends right down at the tips of the toes.

We know that sciatica is usually caused by the compression of one or several of these roots – either by the herniation of an intervertebral disc (so called 'slipped disc'), or, by displacement, or partial dislocation, of one vertebra on another, so pinching the origin of the nerve. So the pain is felt right down the back of the thigh, and leg, maybe even to the toes, rather as a message follows along a telegraph line.

Pain is not the only effect, since when the nerve is very much compressed it stops transmitting at all, and signs of paralysis begin to appear in the leg; this is announced by the onset of the sensation we call 'pins and needles', which is an alarm signal for serious complications, and by weakness of the muscles of the leg.

Of course, acute sciatica such as we have just described – which may occur, as with lumbago, and for the same reasons, after a violent effort such as lifting in a bad position – may well improve and even cure itself after a time, but it may also recur and disable the patient without warning, from time to time.

Various methods are used to treat sciatica; a rest in bed, perhaps on traction; strong analgesic drugs; injections round the nerve; a manipulation to free the compressed nerve root; and as a last resort, an operation.

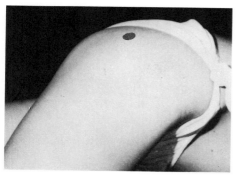

In the meantime, massaging the appropriate points can bring about considerable relief. These are, firstly, the painful points which you can find along the course of the nerve; and secondly, a more specific point, which is equally effective for all pain in the lower limb.

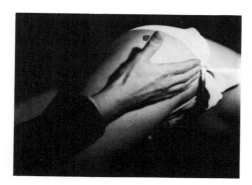

This point is situated on the outerside of the buttock, just behind the bulge which constitutes the top of the long thigh bone, the femur, and which is known scientifically as the trochanter, as in the diagram opposite.

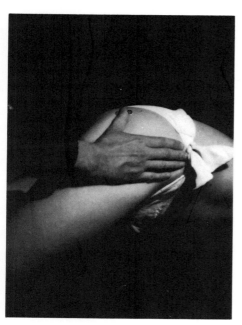

A good way of finding this point is to lie the patient down on his healthy side with the affected leg half bent, and place your four fingers along the iliac crest. If the thumb is then held at right angles, as in the photograph, it will exactly indicate the point.

Breast pain

Women's breasts are vulnerable areas of the body which are easily injured, and may become painful; they are also liable to certain malfunctions and diseases. Women are very aware of the possibility of developing breast cancer; many have learnt to conduct self-examination for lumps, and do so regularly, especially if their breasts are painful. Pain does not necessarily indicate danger, however. During the menstrual cycle, breasts swell up and go down again to a varying degree depending on the individual. And this may be very painful, in the same way as inflammation of the nipples, and the small cysts which are common at the time of the menopause can be; and mothers who are breast feeding their babies may find that this is painful also.

Of course, if there is something abnormal in the breast, you must consult a doctor without delay, but in the meantime there is no harm in relieving your discomfort with the two massage points, which are, in fact, some distance away.

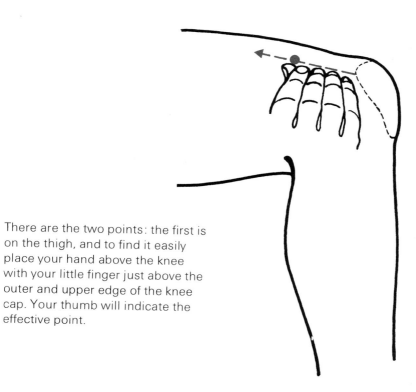

There are the two points: the first is
on the thigh, and to find it easily
place your hand above the knee
with your little finger just above the
outer and upper edge of the knee
cap. Your thumb will indicate the
effective point.

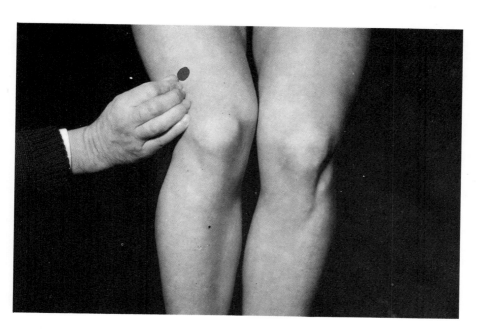

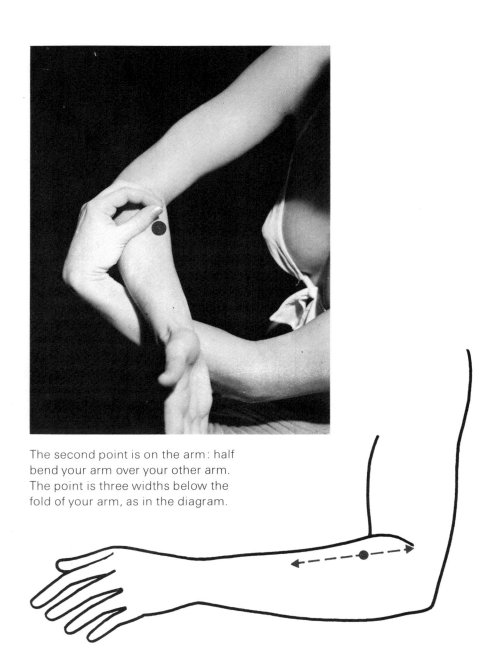

The second point is on the arm: half
bend your arm over your other arm.
The point is three widths below the
fold of your arm, as in the diagram.

Sexuality

In the West, research into sexuality, for so long a 'taboo' subject, started only relatively recently. According to Freud, of course, our early sexual development is fundamental to the formation of our personality and our adult behaviour.

For the Chinese, however, sexual energy is part of our general human energy, which, together with food and the air we breathe, is essential for building and maintaining our vital strength. So maintaining sexual energy is, for the Chinese, not just an agreeable pastime, but is also seen as being a pressing need for the general health of the body.

Impotence in the male

Many factors are thought to contribute to impotence. There may be a physical cause such as genital abnormality, or a serious infection; but these days impotence is far more often due to the strain and tiredness caused by modern city life, or to psychological problems which may have to be traced back to a forgotten episode, maybe in childhood or adolescence. Impotence in middle-aged professional men is a well recognized condition, and may be taken as a sign of the extent to which they are preoccupied with their occupations, and have time for nothing else. A good relaxing holiday is often a remarkable cure.

For a speedier and less expensive approach to the problem, there are two points which are very effective. The first is on the abdomen, exactly halfway between the navel and the pubic bone.

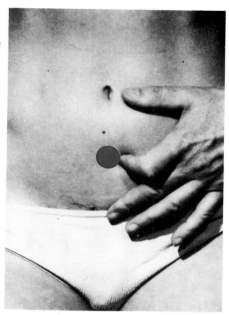

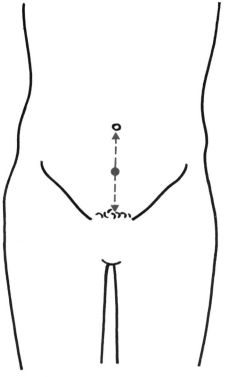

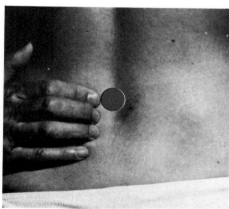

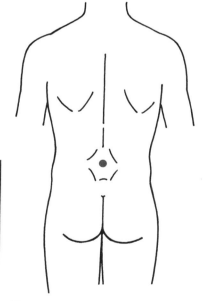

The second is on the back, on the vertebral column, four finger widths above the large bone known as the sacrum.

Frigidity and infertility in women

For the Chinese, frigidity, the inability to feel sexually aroused and satisfied, is synonymous with sterility, and is thought to affect the woman's ability to conceive.

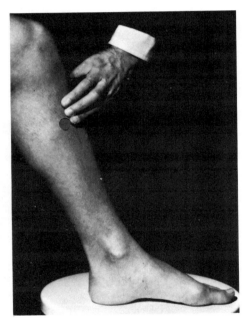

There are two massage points. The first point is situated on the inside of the leg. Find the upper end of the tibia, near the knee. Moving your hand down the side, you will feel a bend, and the point is three finger widths below this, as in the diagram.

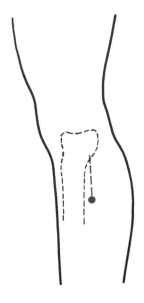

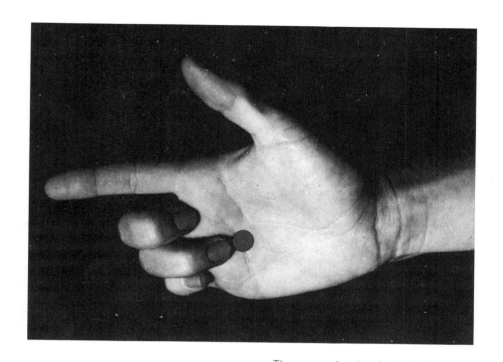

The second point, in the hollow of the hand, is easy to find. It is on the palm, where the finger bends on to the head line.

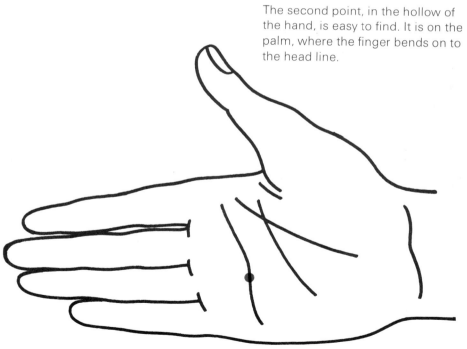

Faintness

Fainting and loss of consciousness may be caused by a number of things. Some are serious, for example cardiac causes, and you should consult a doctor. You may feel faint after sudden and intense physical pain such as severe renal colic or a coronary thrombosis. But in the vast majority of cases, the situation, while dramatic, is less serious. You may, for example feel faint after hearing some bad news, or again you may have low blood pressure, and be liable to feel faint when suddenly sitting or standing up after lying down for some time. Or you may be one of those people who have a liability to fainting attacks, because of slowing of the heart rate.

Whatever the cause, you will need to have a means of counteracting this fainting feeling.

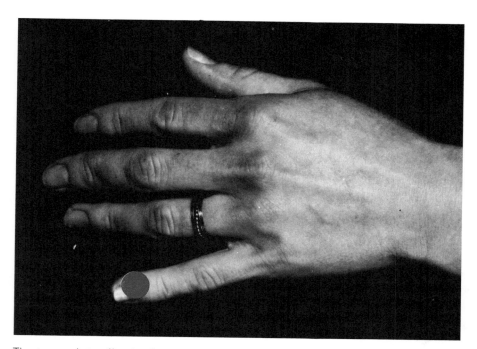

The two points effective for faintness are on the little fingers on the ring finger side, at the right angle formed by a line along the base of the fingernail with a vertical line down the side of the nail.

You will need to lie the patient down and massage forcefully, and if you are applying the pressure to yourself, you can do this lying down and using your folded thumb.

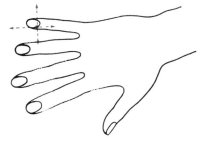

Forceful massage revives the patient and avoids all possibility of loss of consciousness.

Headache

Headaches are perhaps more common than aches in any other part of the body. There are a large number of causes, from flu to indigestion, to a brain tumour; not to mention eyestrain, or any number of psychosomatic causes.

A careful medical examination is necessary to diagnose the real trouble, but in the meantime relief can be provided by one of three points, depending on the exact site of the headache.

1. Headache on the forehead or temples, on one or both sides.
2. Headache on the nape of the neck and back of the head.
3. Headache in the skull, and generally all over.

1. Headache on the forehead or temples, on one or both sides.

The effective point is situated on the wrist, where the pulse is taken, but a little higher. To locate it accurately, on the right hand for example, hold your right hand flat, palm upwards and thumb out; lock your right thumb over your left hand thumb, and with the three smaller fingers on your left hand wrapped around your right hand, you will find that your index finger held straight will point exactly to the point.

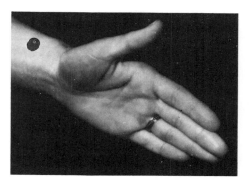

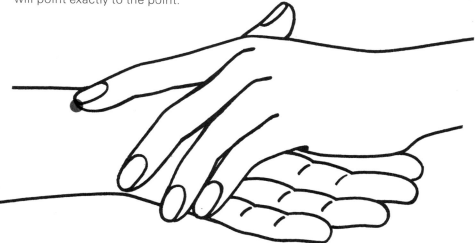

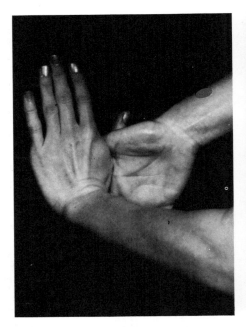

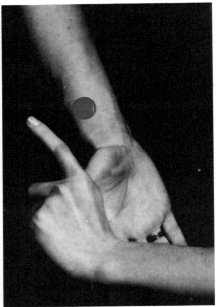

Note, however, that if your entire forehead aches, you should stimulate the point on both wrists. If only one side hurts, stimulate the point on the opposite hand; that is, if the headache is on the right side, stimulate the left wrist; for a headache on the left side, use the right wrist.

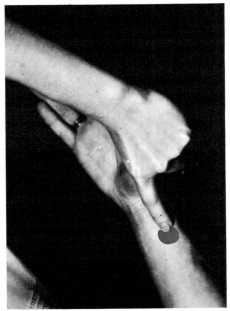

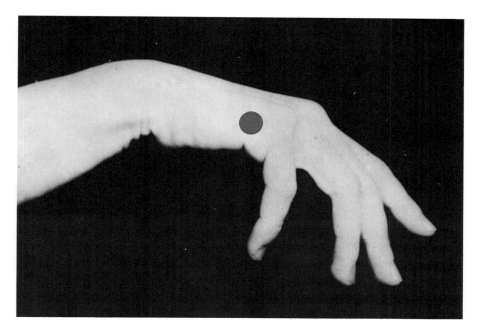

2. Headache on the nape of the neck and back of the head

The effective point is once again on the hand, on the little finger side. Half bend your hand, and you will notice the 'head line' crease; your finger extends into it, and you will be able to feel the bone known as the fifth metacarpal.

You will feel slight pain on bending the hand in this way, and you should stimulate at that point. Again, stimulate the right hand side if your pain is on the left side and vice versa.

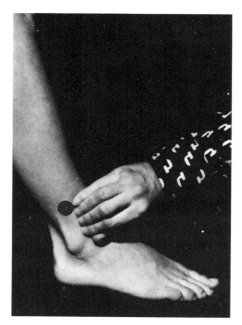

3. Headache in the skull, and generally all over

For this variety of migrane, you can use all the points which apply to 1 and 2, together with the point known as 'bladder'. This is situated at the bottom of the leg, on the outer side, in a small hollow on the front of the long thin bone called the fibula. To find it exactly, with your thumb and fingers together, place the end of your little finger on the protrusion of the ankle bone, and your thumb will indicate the point, as in the diagram.

Massage these two points with your hands crossed, right hand on the left leg, and vice versa.

A last word about headaches: the Chinese have always felt that acupuncture is so effective in treating headaches, that its failure can only indicate that something is very wrong, for example a brain tumour.

Stage fright

The student taking an exam, the singer walking on to the stage, the preacher in his pulpit or the lecturer in the lecture hall – all suffer from 'nerves': a dry mouth and throat, a rapid pulse and a throbbing forehead, and difficulty controlling the voice.

Everyone has felt stage fright at some time or another. But for some people it can be a real disability which can restrict their activities, inhibit their development, and prevent them from fulfilling their ambitions. So it is well worth knowing of an effective point which can fight these effects.

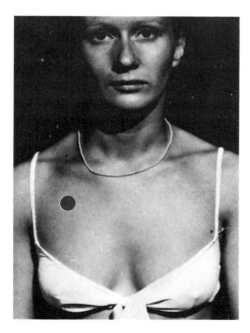 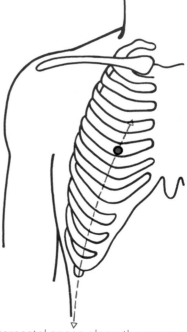

This point, which is also effective for mental and physical shocks or frights, may be stimulated through the clothing. It is high on the right side of the chest, four finger widths above the right nipple, in the second intercostal space along the mammary meridian. Stimulate it forcefully, and you will calm down and feel relaxed.

This point was regularly stimulated by Napoleon, as pictures show.

121

Intestinal worms

You may well ask how stimulation of tiny points on the skin surface can possibly rid the body of those undesirable inhabitants of the lower intestine: worms. And yet, Chinese traditional and practical experience have confirmed that acupuncture is an excellent treatment for this condition. Once again, we cannot help asking how this can be possible.

We might suggest that stimulation triggers off intestinal contractions, which expel the worms. But neither clinical experience, nor recordings of intestinal movement have shown this to be the case. We are left thinking that stimulation of the point in some way modifies the environment of the intestine, so that life becomes impossible for the parasites. Besides, the author of this book has observed that stimulation of this point has often eradicated cutaneous mycoses (that is, fungal infections of the skin, such as athlete's foot).

So this point appears to arouse the body's defence mechanisms against parasites.

The point is situated at the end of
the little toe, at the right angle
formed in the intersection of the two
lines, one along the base, and the
other along the outside, of the nail.

Facial care

Coquettes in the past have been criticized for spending hours in front of a mirror. And yet some people argue that beauty is a gift which ought to be cared for; but while the surface of the body depends on the quality of its foundations, there are numerous methods of caring for the skin, and virtually none at all which are concerned with the facial muscles. Whilst we maintain our biceps and exercise our abdominal muscles, we neglect our many tiny facial muscles; those, as Darwin wrote, that express our emotions, our laughter and smiles; but which, when relaxed, betray our wrinkles, and reveal our sagging ageing features.

So acupuncture finds its place in beauty care. Regular stimulation of points on the face tones up muscles, and delays the appearance of ageing.

There are several acupunture points
on the face: we have chosen six,
three on each side.

The first is on the forehead, two
finger widths beyond the outer end
of the eyebrow, and four finger
widths above it; the second is on
the underside of the cheek bone,
facing the nose; the third is situated
exactly at the corner of the mouth,
one finger width along from where
the lips meet.

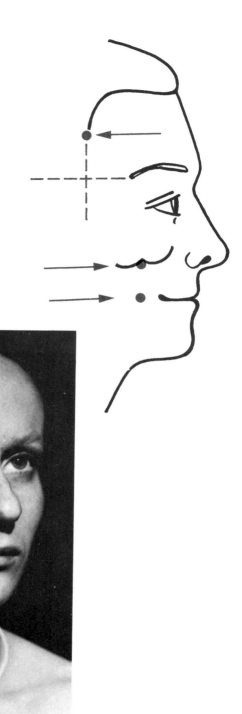

Vomiting

It is beneficial to vomit if you are ridding your body of toxic substances or bad food which may cause trouble once it has passed into the intestines. But vomiting is unpleasant, and in some cases can be dangerous, since it causes loss of fluid and essential mineral salts. So it is usually wise to relieve yourself of this symptom, since it may aggravate your condition.

Even if we benefit from paying for our over indulgence, it is as well to put a stop to the vomiting at the stage where the stomach is empty and yet continues to contract, bringing up only acid, phlegm, and possibly blood.

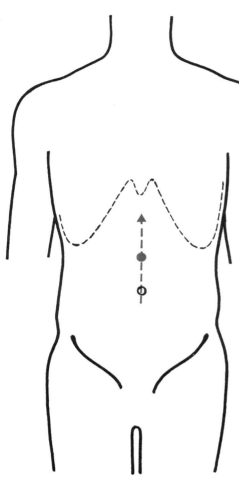

One massage point is very effective.
This point is situated on the upper
part of the wall of the abdomen,
along the meridian line, halfway
between the navel and the
protrusion at the bottom of the
sternum.

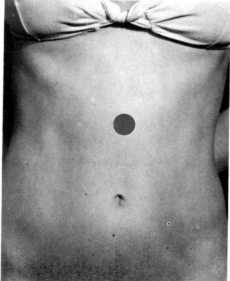

Aching eyes

Your eyes may feel painful for a number of reasons: a blow, a speck of dust, or an infection such as conjunctivitis. There are also more serious causes, such as iritis or glaucoma, to mention the major ones, which endanger the vision. For this reason, you should always be extremely careful if your eyes start to ache, and consult a doctor as soon as possible. He will conduct a careful examination of the eyes, in particular the back of the eye, the retina, and the nerve which collects the visual images and transmits them to the brain; he will also measure the tension of the eye. Hypertension indicates glaucoma, which may destroy vision within hours. But meantime we suffer, and perhaps can scarcely see, since the other eye shuts also protectively as a reflex.

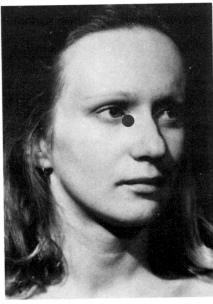

One point can bring rapid relief. This point is situated close to the healthy eye, near the inside corner.
Massage the left point firmly to treat the right eye, and vice versa. If both eyes are inflamed, use both points simultaneously.

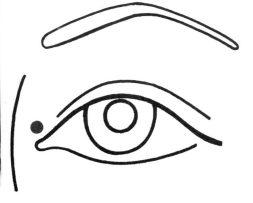

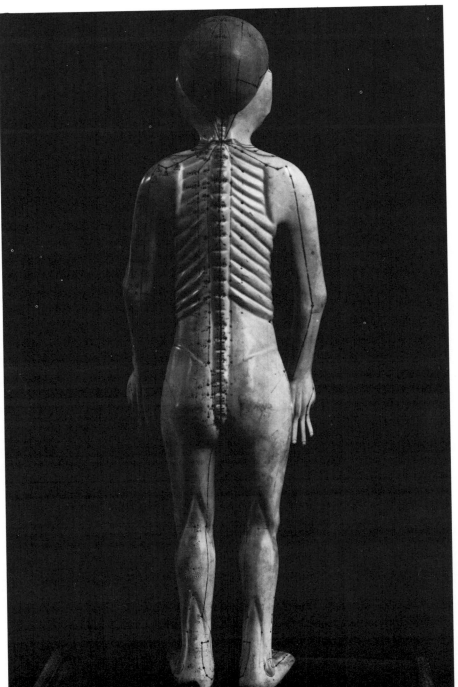

photo Roger Viollet

The Scientific Explanation

Is there a scientific basis for the use of acupuncture? This question is frequently asked by patients and doubting doctors. There is little difficulty in producing an impressive and often surprising list of therapeutic successes. But therapeutic successes are not regarded by the doctors as indisputable proof, since it can be argued that these results are only the fruit of the imagination, or that the very fact of the acupuncturist's presence sets up a dependence relationship which persuades the patient of the good effect the treatment is having. In other words, acupuncture is merely a 'placebo', or if it works in any other way, it is by 'suggestion'. Ever since acupuncture appeared in the West, doctors who became enthusiastic about it tried desperately to provide scientific proof of its method of action, and yet 'scientific proof' is a Western concept, which has to be obtained under laboratory conditions in the same way as proof is obtained for all Western medicine.

Well, there are now numerous proofs. Firstly, indirect, but unsatisfactory, proofs; these are instrumental measurements taken on healthy and unhealthy patients by physiological or biological methods analysed afterwards. There are too many of these results, since sets of figures obtained from needles can be shuffled about and made to prove anything.

Results obtained during the course of acupuncture have, therefore, to be scrupulously recorded, and results examined and analysed in relation to their effects on four systems of the body: effects on blood composition; on the functioning of the heart; on respiration; and on the digestive system. Firstly, it has been shown that stimulation of certain acupuncture points causes the blood to become enriched; a considerable increase in the number of red blood corpuscles appears two or three minutes after

Japanese medicine: acupuncture doll (seen from the back)

stimulation. Secondly, patients who have disturbed heart rhythms show a marked improvement on the electrocardiogram after acupuncture. The heartbeat becomes regular both in quantity and in quality, and this improvement is observed on the electrocardiogram. Thirdly, respiratory function has been analysed using spirometers, which register the working of the lungs, and a marked improvement has been observed, particularly in asthmatic patients, where bronchial spasms die down gradually under the action of the acupuncture needles.

But fourthly, in France recently, the most spectacular results have been obtained during observations on the digestive system. The working of the digestive organs has been recorded electronically, using electrodes similar to those of an electrocardiograph, but placed on the patient's abdomen. From these, the movements of the stomach and the intestines, called 'peristalsis', have been recorded. When peristalsis has been considerable, and it sometimes becomes very painful, causing colic, the application of acupuncture needles to the front of the abdomen has brought about considerable reduction of activity and a general calming of the system.

All this is evidence that acupuncture works. We can see that acupuncture, in the form of massage, or the insertion of needles, acts on the organs, but this evidence does not explain how or why it works.

Although the medical profession in the West is prepared to use certain methods of treatment which have been found to work, in spite of the fact that they do not know the reason why, and this particularly applies to certain forms of psychiatric treatment, there is a surprising resistance to the use of acupuncture, which has also been shown to work, but for which, until very recently, it has not been possible to provide a scientific explanation. This is why it has been of great importance to investigate the actual mechanism by which acupuncture acts on the body.

Recent research in laboratories in the Western world, in France, Scotland, Canada and the United States in particular, has produced a number of discoveries that throw light on the way in which acupuncture and even pressure of the fingers may produce their effect. We shall describe these in the chapters that follow, in relation to the various levels with which they are concerned.

The Mechanism of Action at Skin Level

Let us start at the surface of the body, with evidence for the action at skin level. But how can we register at skin level proof that something particular is happening at the points and meridians of acupuncture? In the following way. For a long time it has been observed that 'something was happening at these points and along the meridian network'. But this is what we have in fact been saying all along. Stimulation of the point brings about a change in the pain sensitivity, a raising of the pain threshold, so that it becomes different from that of neighbouring tissues.

For some time also, electric currents have been administered at the acupuncture points, and it has been observed that electric sensation is felt more intensely by the subject at these points than in adjacent areas, to the extent that the pain was felt to be unbearable in the former, while scarcely any at all was felt in the latter. This effect has now been thoroughly investigated with the consent of some patients. The skin of the immediate underlying area has been removed and examined under the microscope to see if there is any sort of nerve terminal or other specialized structure present. Disappointingly, nothing was detected, but research in another direction has produced more rewarding results.

Doctors have spent years recording electrical currents and resistance at the acupuncture points and meridian lines, and comparing these with other parts of the skin; but until recently all such results were open to the criticism that the smallest amount of pressure on the skin will alter resistance, and this, of course, includes the pressure exerted by the recording electrodes themselves.

In New York, however, Dr Becker and his associates have been using teflon, rather than metal, electrodes; these have the advantage that they exert minimal pressure, thus eliminating error as far as possible. Using this new technique, it has been found that electrical resistance and conductivity are different if measured between acupuncture points and meridians, and other areas of the skin.

Electrical conductivity is greatest at the points, and decreases sharply in surrounding areas. There is an oval area around each point, away from which conductivity decreases gradually. Thus there is direct evidence of the existence of the points themselves.

Similarly, it has been shown that conductivity is greater along the meridian lines than elsewhere. Becker and his colleagues placed two electrodes a few centimetres apart, along one of the meridians, and set up a parallel pair one centimetre away from them. Electric current passed far more readily along the meridian line than along its parallel. Consequently, *it is certain that there are specific electrical properties at the points, and along the meridians, that are different from those of the surrounding tissues.*

These researches have been the starting point of new hypotheses which are currently being investigated. The general theory of Becker and his colleagues is that there is a nervous system in the skin which developed earlier and is more primitive than the central nervous system, probably a remnant from an earlier embryonic stage. The human embryo, as it develops, passes through a stage when it is similar to an amphibian, or a fish with gills. At this stage, before the definitive central nervous system has formed, a primitive nervous network appears, which persists at skin level. It is a system concerned with the defence and growth of the skin, and it comes into action throughout a person's life; for example, when the skin is injured. It is suggested that acupuncture acts through this system, and that the system acts as a transmission network, with the meridian lines functioning as cables, and the nuclei, where the information is at a maximum, acting as centres which amplify and reinforce the amount of energy in the system.

It is astonishing to see how this modern American theory ties in exactly with the Chinese concept of the *acupuncture points as energy junctions which relay and reinforce energy along the meridian lines, and which organize the passage of this energy through the skin towards the organs and the central nervous system.*

There is an extraordinary similarity between these two theories, which are four thousand years apart, and we shall find this similarity again when we come to consider the mode of action of acupuncture on the spinal cord and the central nervous system.

The Mechanism of Action at spinal cord level

To understand the theory of how acupuncture influences the sensation of pain in the spinal cord it is first necessary to know something about the anatomy and physiology of pain, and to learn a little medical terminology. The classical conception of the transmission of pain was very simple. The earlier researchers knew that there were nerve terminals in the skin and the various organs, and they thought that all types of nerve fibres could transmit all types of sensation, whether cold, warmth, touch or pain. These nerve fibres terminate in the back part of the spinal cord, in the area known as the 'posterior horn'. From here the pain message ascends to the brain, and it is in the brain that the message is identified as being painful; it becomes 'pain'. But this classical theory goes back many years, and there have been recent and very important developments.

It is now known that there are two types of nerves concerned with the transmission of pain sensation. The first group, known as A-delta fibres, are relatively thick, and insulated; the second group, the C-fibres, are much finer, and are not insulated. Impulses are transmitted much more quickly in the A-delta fibres than in the C-fibres, with the result that when we hurt

134

ourselves we feel first, almost instantaneously, a sharp pain sensation, and then after a second or so a duller but more prolonged pain. This is because the actual sensation is being transmitted to the brain at two speeds through the two types of nerve fibre, and is being experienced separately, a little while apart. By inserting electrodes into the actual nerve fibres, it has been possible to record the electrical signals passing along them, and to show the difference of speed with which the signals are transmitted. All these nerves terminate, as we have mentioned, in the posterior horn of the spinal cord, in a region called, because of its jelly-like appearance, the *substantia gelatinosa*. In this region they make contact with cells which are connected, through the long nerve tracts which run up the spinal cord, with the brain. In the *substantia gelatinosa* region also, it has long been known that there are large numbers of small nerve cells, but until recently it did not seem that they had any purpose.

It is an everyday experience that pain perception varies greatly not only between different people, but in the same person from time to time, depending on all sorts of circumstances, such as distraction of attention from the pain itself by something of greater interest. We have all heard of the sportsman who has finished the game in spite of injury, and has been oblivious to the pain of a deep cut or fracture until it has suddenly started to hurt when the game came to an end and his attention was no longer diverted from it. An explanation of this and other variations in pain sensation was proposed in 1965 by two doctors, one British, and the other American, Professors Wall and Melzack. They suggested, as a result of much research into the small cells in the *substantia gelatinosa,* that they acted as a 'pain gate', switching on and off the transmission of impulses from the pain nerves into the cells of the spinal cord. This has become known as the *gate theory* of pain. Wall and Melzack suggest that the pain perception mechanism was influenced partly by signals coming down the spinal cord from the brain and controlling the small switching cells, and partly by nerve impulses reaching the *substantia gelatinosa* through a different group of nerve fibres coming mainly from the skin and the muscles, called the A-beta fibres. These A-beta fibres are also quite thick and insulated, and they end in the region of the small switching cells in the *substantia gelatinosa*. They carry the signals for such sensations as touch, rubbing, vibration, pressure and temperature, and if the signals are very frequent and intense they cause, to a greater or lesser extent, the switching off of the pain signals. Conversely, if there is not much activity in the A-beta fibres, the pain fibres are switched on. It is not suggested, of course, that a physical gate exists. The word 'gate' is used metaphorically in the same way as it is used in electronics, to signify the switching on and off of a circuit by means of electrical signals.

This gate theory explains how it is possible for pain to be disregarded either by a conscious decision in the brain, or because the brain attention is so intensely concentrated on something else, that is sends switching-off signals down the spinal cord. It also explains how pain sensations can be affected by things happening at skin level. Rubbing the skin when one is hurt, or warming it, sends signals along the A-beta fibres which switch off some or all of the pain connections in the *substantia gelatinosa*.

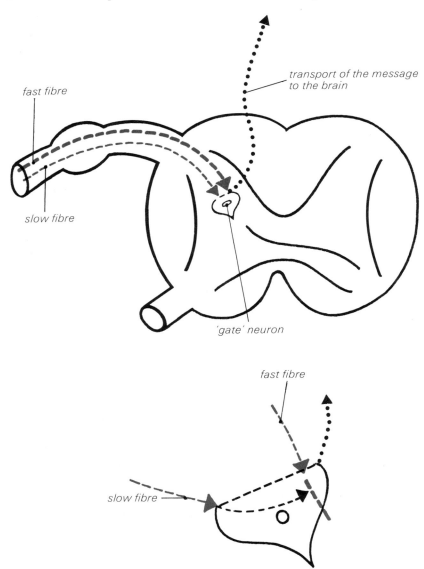

fast fibre

transport of the message
to the brain

slow fibre

'gate' neuron

fast fibre

slow fibre

And this, of course, at spinal cord level, is how we now think acupuncture works. It is beginning to be shown that some of the A-beta fibres terminate in the skin at the principal acupuncture points; so stimulation of one of these points will trigger off a continuous signal to the spinal cord, so 'shutting the gate' and blocking the passage of painful sensations to the brain.

This, in part, explains how surgical operations can be performed using acupuncture instead of conventional anaesthesia. By stimulating the appropriate point, according to Chinese tradition, before, during, and after the operation, painful sensations are blocked, and the surgeon can operate in a tranquil atmosphere, with all the advantages for him and for the patient.

What can be done in surgery may also be useful in medical conditions, including those that have been described in the preceeding pages of this book.

The Mechanism of Action at brain level

One of the most recent and exciting discoveries about the way in which the brain works has been shown to be closely related to the effects of acupuncture, and it is a strange and surprising coincidence that the research was originally concerned with something apparently quite different. Scientists were trying to discover how morphine, a drug known and used to relieve pain for the last three or four thousand years, worked in the brain, and, using a new and powerful research technique, they made a very unexpected discovery.

Before we go on to describe this, however, it is necessary for us to say something about the structure of the nervous tissue in the brain, and how messages pass through it.

The Structure of the brain

Like the rest of the body, the brain is made up of cells, which are the building blocks of living matter. In the brain there are several varieties of these cells. There are some which have the purpose of providing support, defence and nutrition; but we are interested here in the most important cells, the real nerve cells – the neurones. Here, again, we must use some medical terminology. As with all cells, the neurones are composed of a nucleus and a body – which we call protoplasm. But certain of the neurones are different and distinctive in that they have one long prolongation, a long filament called an axon, and a number of much shorter filaments called dendrites, sticking out from them.

To get an idea of what one of these neurones is like, imagine a lamp standard with hairs growing out of the top of the lamp. The standard represents the axon, the lamp is the cell itself, and the hairs represent the dendrites.

Now the axons are actually the nerve fibres that we spoke about in the last section. They may be very long indeed. In the sciatic nerve, which is the longest nerve in the body, they are anything up to three feet long, depending on how tall the person is. The actual neurones, the cells, of the sciatic nerve, are in the spinal cord, but the axons extend as far as the tips of the toes, and transmit messages to and from them. Messages, or nervous impulses, as they are called, pass up and down the axons like an electric current, by a method known as depolarization. When the impulse reaches the neurone it has to be passed on to the next cell in the chain, for transmission up the spinal cord and to the brain. This is the function of the short, fine filaments, the dendrites. They make contact with the surface of the next cell, and under the microscope they look a bit like the tentacles of an octopus attached to its prey.

But the method of transmission of the impulse from one cell to the next one is quite different from the way it passes up the axon. We have seen that in the axon it flows up like an electric current. From one cell to the next, however, it is transmitted by means of a chemical substance produced in the first neurone and passed by means of the dendrites to the second. A very complicated mechanism is concerned in the production of this chemical messenger by the first neurone, and the means by which it is released and sent off to make contact with the second neurone. When it arrives there it is identified by and attaches itself to a special site on the cell surface, rather as a boat enters a harbour and ties up at its place of anchorage. The effect of this chemical reaching its special site has been compared with the effect of inserting and turning a key in a lock; if it is the correct key, the door is opened. If it is the wrong key, the lock jams. In the neurone, when the 'right key' is turned in the lock, the receiving cell is stimulated, and the message passed onwards, again electrically; and the chemical messenger, its task completed, is rapidly destroyed.

For about thirty years, only one chemical messenger was known to exist. Then modern methods of analysis revealed another, and then more. At the present time, a number of different chemical messengers, so called 'transmitters', have been found – adrenalin, serotonin, dopamine, gamma aminobutyric acid – some of these stimulate the brain, others depress some of its functions, and there is now growing evidence that they may be concerned in the causation of mental illness if they are present in abnormal quantities.

The consequences of these discoveries are staggering. The nervous cells are really glands capable of secreting chemical substances, and often sending them off some distance; and not all cells secrete the same substance. This varies, depending on the region of the brain and its special functions – as one might say, depending on the message, so the 'messenger' changes.

Natural drugs

After these very exciting discoveries, scientists moved on to thinking that this junction between neurones might not only be a zone of great activity, but also an area of great sensitivity, susceptible to injury or poisoning. As we have said, inserting the wrong key jams the lock, and a number of drugs are now known to act like the 'wrong key' at these junctions; for example, the aerosol insecticides, and curare.

Some researchers, then, considered the effects of various intoxicating substances, some quite dangerous, and not used medicinally as drugs, so called 'psychedelic' substances; and, with the object of helping addicts, work has been done also to investigate the action of narcotic drugs on the central nervous system, in particular, 'hard' drugs such as opium, and its derivative morphine. Using radioactive methods, it has been found that morphine is accepted by certain nerve cells in the brain. These neurones have at their surface specific sites to which morphine molecules can attach themselves – once again the notion of anchorage that we mentioned above. When this was first discovered it created great excitement among scientists. It was thought to be extraordinary that nature could foresee that a vegetable substance, from a flower, the poppy, would enter into contact with the nervous system to the extent that its arrival was perfectly well prepared for. Then came the flash of inspiration. If such an alien substance was accepted, it must be similar to a natural production secreted by the brain itself. As so often nowdays, demonstration followed quickly upon the idea, and within a few months, at Aberdeen University, and La Jolla University in California, a series of chemical messengers in the brain, chemically very similar to morphine, were discovered. These have been called endorphines, or natural morphines, and they have the same effect as the drug morphine, that is to say, they suppress pain. They appear to work by blocking the transmission of pain impulses from one neurone to another, like the 'wrong key' in the lock.

There have now been discovered a number of these substances, all rather similar chemically, which are known to have a calming, or even a euphoric effect, producing optimism, or even joy, according to their chemical structure and the place of production either in the brain, the pituitary gland, and so on.

Role of acupuncture

What has all this to do with acupuncture? A Canadian scientist, Professor Pomeranz of Toronto, made the crucial discovery: acupuncture liberated these very endorphines. The idea of looking for this effect came to him – so he tells us – when he saw the way the Chinese use acupuncture before surgery; they stimulate the acupuncture point for at least twenty minutes before starting to operate, and this is the time necessary for the formation of the chemical substance, the endorphine. Pomeranz gives these proofs:

(1) Cerebro-spinal fluid, the fluid which bathes the brain and spinal cord, taken from a subject anaesthetized by acupuncture, transmits this sedative effect to another who is not acupunctured. This is evidence that there is a chemical substance present in the cerebro-spinal fluid of a subject treated with acupuncture with effects which may be transmitted by injection.

(2) Using electrodes attached to the brain of an animal, Pomeranz registered the reactions of the neurones to pain. The reactions are signalled by a certain number of 'blips' on the trace. These 'blips', signifying the transmission of painful impulses, diminish and then stop completely when the acupuncture point is stimulated, even though pain is still being provoked.

(3) Finally Pomeranz used a chemical substance which blocks the action of morphine, and of endorphine also, in the brain. This is a morphine antidote, 'naloxone', a 'wrong key', which, attaching itself to the morphine site on the surface of the neurones, prevents morphine from producing its usual action. Naloxone also has the effect of preventing acupuncture from relieving pain, and it also reverses the pain relief already produced by acupuncture if it is injected afterwards. This is virtually proof that acupuncture acts by stimulating the production of endorphines.

But Pomeranz goes further. He deduces from this that prolonged action demands similarly prolonged stimulation, from twenty minutes to an hour, and, whichever the method of stimulation – injection, electricity or simple massage – the result obtained has an identical effect on the pain. Isn't this the very justification for the methods described in this book?

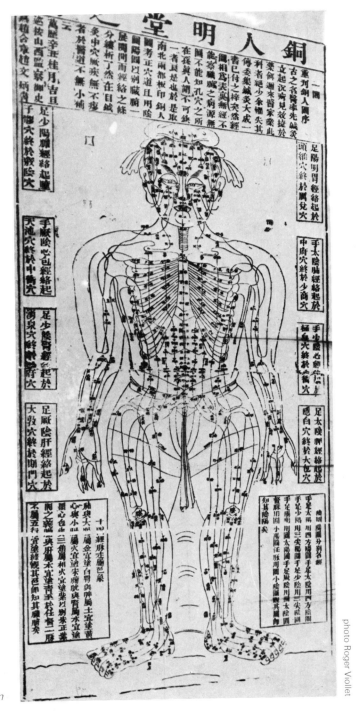

Chinese Medicine:
Acupuncture diagram

photo Roger Viollet

Conclusion

You are now ready to provide relief for yourself if you are suffering from one of over fifty common ailments described in this book.

As we have said more than once, we are talking about temporary relief; for full diagnosis and treatment you should consult your doctor. But at least you can abate the pain and prevent it from getting worse. And perhaps your observations, of which we are always glad to learn, can help advance a branch of medicine which has strong connections with the past, and holds rich promise for the future.

We will be more than satisfied if we have aroused your curiosity, and enabled you to relieve some troublesome complaints.

Ancient China
Statuette showing the affected part of the patient's body.
Women would send these to their doctors.

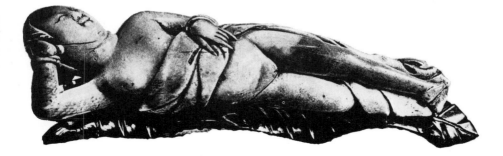